Health Metamorphosis

Dori Luneski, R.N., N.D.
American Wellness Company

KENDALL/HUNT PUBLISHING COMPANY
4050 Westmark Drive   Dubuque, Iowa 52002

Cover artwork and interior illustrations:
Rebecca Grace Jones

Copyright © 1997 by American Wellness Company

Library of Congress Catalog Card Number: 97-72123.

ISBN 0-7872-3650-0

All rights reserved. No part of this publication may be reproduced, stored in a retrieval system, or transmitted, in any form or by any means, electronic, mechanical, photocopying, recording, or otherwise, without the prior written permission of the copyright owner.

Printed in the United States of America
10 9 8 7 6 5 4 3 2 1

I DEDICATE THIS BOOK

To...

Robert H. Schuller *from the Crystal Cathedral Ministries, who strengthened my awareness that I am God's child and He has a plan for me.*

To...

my sons **Bob and Dan,** *who I have learned to understand, and who have learned to understand me.*

To...

my dearest friend, **Charles Miller,** *who is one of God's nicest people.*

And to...

Marijane Thompson, *whose excellence in everything she does makes all my hard days easier. Without her valuable assistance, the completion of this book would have been immeasurably more difficult.*

DISCLAIMER

HEALTH METAMORPHOSIS is not intended to treat disease, in any way interfere with diagnostic procedures or treatment by any medical practitioner, or be construed as medical advice. This book may seem controversial to some; it is not intended to satisfy modern science. The opinions herein are strictly those of the author. The "first do no harm" recommendations in this book are meant to be guidelines to assist the body to work at optimal performance, or heal itself if possible. Even in the face of serious illness, the principles of wellness should not be ignored. The author urges anyone having a health concern to see a licensed practitioner for evaluation. The application of any concepts in this book without the consent of a licensed practitioner is not encouraged; however, it is your constitutional right to decide how you wish to treat your body. The author and the publisher assume no liability for the implementation of any material presented.

TABLE OF CONTENTS

Foreword	ix
Why You Should Read This Book	xi
Introduction	xiii

Chapter 1
POSITIVE THINKING IS POSSIBILITY THINKING ----- 1

How to Resolve a Problem	5
The Three Ways to Program the Subconscious	12
Pay-offs for Hanging On to Illness	13
Mindtraps Keep You Locked in the Past	14
Ways to Enhance Your Potential	16
Basic Personality Groups	25
Be in Charge of Your Personal Development	28
Now Go For It!	35

Chapter 2
NUTRITION ----- 37

The Villains	39
The Heroes	53
Here are Some Facts on Protein Choices	64
Breakfast or Brunch Suggestions	71
Lunch Suggestions	74
Spirulina - Vegetable Drink	76
HELP for Shopping	79

Chapter 3
DIGESTION ----- 83

A Walk Through the Digestive Process	84
Are You Ready to Improve Your Digestion?	88
Some Supplements That Aid Digestion	95
Juices that Aid Digestion	97
Herbs For Digestion	97
Acid-Alkaline pH Balance	99
HELP for pH	100
Learn to Love Your Liver	106
Problems from a Malfunctioning Liver	109
Some Foods that Are Bad for the Liver	113
Some Choices that Are Bad for the Liver	113

Diet ----- 115
1, 2, or 3 Day Cleansing ----- 116
Some Foods that Are Good for the Liver ----- 118

Chapter 4
ELIMINATION ----- 123
Natural Parasite Treatments ----- 126
Ways You Accumulate Toxins ----- 128
The Excretory Organs ----- 130
The Major Cause of Toxemia is Constipation ----- 135
Six Requirements for Healthy Elimination ----- 137
Recommendations to Improve Elimination ----- 139
Cleansing Programs with Mucusless Meals ----- 144
Things to Remember in Cleansing ----- 147

Chapter 5
INTERNAL ENERGY ----- 151
How to Develop Enthusiasm to be a Participant in Life ----- 153
Key Points in Achieving Fitness and Prolonging Life Expectancy ----- 159
Exercise Options Have Important Points to Consider ----- 162
Eight Common Sense Health Choices for Circulation ----- 167
Understanding Calcium Absorption ----- 171
Your Lymphatic System ----- 176
Another Form of Energy - Magnetism ----- 179

Summary ----- 183

Recommended Books ----- 191

Recommended References ----- 193

FOREWORD

Sir Arthur Edington once said, "Verily it is easier for a camel to pass through the eye of a needle than for a scientific man to pass through a door, it might be wiser that he should consent to be an ordinary man and walk in, rather than wait till all the difficulties involved in a really scientific ingress are resolved." In *HEALTH METAMORPHOSIS*, Dr. Luneski helps the "health student" walk through the door to an understanding of the principles of emotional, as well as physical health, and well being.

The concepts presented in *HEALTH METAMORPHOSIS* are very appropriate to healing now, and in the Twenty-first Century. Dr. Luneski has clearly shown the relationship between the psyche and spirit to the physical body. She has also provided the reader with a clear understanding of important nutritional concepts that are essential to true wellness. In addition, she has skillfully outlined specific steps to take in putting these principles into action. This book provides a wealth of practical information that will help the serious "student of health" overcome chronic health problems, or simply obtain a higher level of wellness. If the principles in this book are followed, one can truly achieve a positive **health metamorphosis**.

Paul D. Harris, Ph.D

WHY YOU SHOULD READ THIS BOOK

This book is for those who are "sick and tired of being sick and tired". It is for those who seek help and are told that their physical examination and blood chemistry is normal, and are left with unanswered questions as to why they feel so ill. This book is for those who are pacified with a drug because that is what the doctor thinks is expected. The patient is told to come back if symptoms do not improve; by then health may have deteriorated to the point where other medication and/or surgery is recommended.

This book is for those who have been told to eat a "well-balanced diet", but are given minimum information about the laws of wellness. They are left to the mercy of the food industry propaganda. The handouts from medical organizations for dietary advice have such surface information, they only add to the frustration and confusion when nothing seems to help.

This book is for those who have learned that the health-care industry has little to offer for "chronic poor health" except a quick prescription, a pat on the back with no help for your symptoms, or a referral to another doctor with similar disappointing results. A barrage of expensive tests can seem unnecessary; some can have inaccurate information.

There are many people looking for a practical, reasonable method of taking responsibility for their health. This book will provide guidance through the confusion that discourages so many people, who are trying to nurture themselves and their families in a sick world.

Treating disease is complicated; preventing disease is simple. This book simplifies a subject that has been made complicated by modern medicine's treatment of disease, and made confusing by the abundance of preventive medicine's options.

It is true that medically trained people can best treat you for traumatic or acute illnesses. When I broke my hip skiing, I did not ask for a cup of herb tea. However, Robert Mendelsshon, M.D. says in his book *CONFESSIONS OF A MEDICAL HERETIC:*

"I BELIEVE THAT, DESPITE ALL THE SUPER TECHNOLOGY AND ELITE BEDSIDE MANNER THAT'S SUPPOSED TO MAKE YOU FEEL ABOUT AS WELL CARED FOR AS AN ASTRONAUT ON THE WAY TO THE MOON, THE GREATEST DANGER TO YOUR HEALTH IS THE DOCTOR WHO PRACTICES MODERN MEDICINE."

No one is as interested in your health as you are. You alone suffer pain, loss of life enjoyment, premature aging, and untimely death. You go to a modern doctor to feel better *NOW;* too often that is all you get. But, having a symptom relieved is not health. The name of the symptom, the name of the disease is NOT YOUR PROBLEM! Your problem is what *CAUSED* the symptom or disease.

You can read dozens of separate books for knowledge on different health subjects, but my book gives you ALL THE BASIC LAWS OF HEALTH. This is YOUR life. . .you must assume responsibility for preventing disease.

My own illness, trials, struggles, setbacks and successes have enabled me to organize this very practical approach for you, the "health student", to care for yourself and your loved ones. The result will be the enthusiasm that helps you make healthier daily choices. The pay-off for making better decisions is doing what you really want. . .feeling good. . . and enjoying life to the fullest.

                                                  Dori Luneski, R.N., N.D.

INTRODUCTION

Metamorphosis is a change. A slow, wriggling caterpillar pupates; for a time the gray pupa hangs from a twig, while within, a miracle is taking place. The pupa at last splits open, and the butterfly is born, to greet the flowers with beautiful rainbow wings. A human can undergo metamorphosis, too. The cocoon of a sickly body can be broken open, and the healthy, vital new person can escape.

In my life I have undergone a metamorphosis; now people marvel at my excellent health. I was so crippled I could barely function; today at 63, I am vital, full of energy, and feel terrific! People who knew me when I was ill are amazed at my improved health. People meeting me for the first time are impressed with my youthful appearance and vitality. I was fortunate enough to find a constructive path to better health that treated the *CAUSE* of my illness, not just the symptoms. Whether you're ill and want to feel better, or just want to protect your current health, you don't have to search for years, as I did. If you follow THE EIGHT LAWS OF WELLNESS discussed in this book, metamorphosis can happen to you!

Modern medical technology has made it possible for many people to live longer lives. Living a long life, however, should not be your only goal. You should want to be healthy, active, productive and enthusiastic for life in your senior years. The definition of health in Webster's dictionary states: "Physical and mental well-being, soundness, freedom from defeat, pain or disease, normality of mental and physical function". The next line was what I was looking for in the definition, "Health is something different from strength. It is universal good condition." Just because you were able to get up this morning doesn't imply any degree of health! Health is achieved only when you have FREEDOM from symptoms on all levels...physical, emotional, and mental.

In this book we will examine self-health; how you can practice principles of health that allow your body to work at optimum performance, or heal itself if possible. Modern medicine practitioners best understand the complexities of the human body, but everyone should have a basic understanding of how to make choices for his or her well being. *HEALTH METAMORPHOSIS* will teach you how what you eat, think, and do affects your health.

▯ ▯ ▯ ▯ ▯ ▯

My path to good health has been a long one. I realize now that the harm I was doing to my body didn't immediately make me sick, and the good health practices I later learned didn't cure me in a week. With such a slow process, you don't see immediate results from any action, whether health-building or health-destroying. What started as a few annoying symptoms took years to develop into debilitating illness.

My first symptom at age 25 was pain in my ribs. I didn't realize it at the time, but that was the beginning of gradually deteriorating health that 20 years later left me nearly an invalid. It started when a doctor treated my symptoms with an anti-inflammatory drug. When I moved to Eugene, Oregon, a doctor continued my treatment for the same unresolved distress. For four years, I was treated with a variety of medications. Each symptom was treated separately; I was referred to specialists, each of whom was involved in only a narrow field of medicine. None of these physicians suggested looking for the *CAUSE* of my complaints. Some medications did help suppress the symptoms, but I never felt well.

As I got sicker, I developed a disease one of my doctors called Polymyositis, an inflammatory muscle disease. This diagnosis was not the beginning of new hope; in fact, I was about to embark on a 12-year nightmare. In the first year, my doctors prescribed so many drugs that charts were necessary to keep it all straight. Some medications produced side effects; other medications were required to counteract the side effects.

Our society has learned to accept the end result of poor health and not ask doctors to explain what *CAUSED* their illness; and in many cases the doctors may not even know. My doctors quickly discouraged questions; they did not encourage me to take part in decisions concerning my health, but to "trust them". Symptoms were treated. . .causes were ignored.

My doctors *NEVER* recommended supplements. "Just eat a good diet", I was told by one doctor after another. I ate what is generally regarded as a "good diet". That diet is based on our society's standards, and that meant low fiber, too little raw food, too much cooked and processed food, excess of mucous forming and poorly digested red meat and dairy products, high fat, refined sugar, junk food, and additives.

None of the doctors discussed the details of what a health-building diet should be. I am a Registered Nurse, but even in the nursing program, the laws of wellness were not emphasized.

I had been taught as a nurse to follow directions, and to trust what the doctors said was correct. Despite being cared for with modern technology's finest equipment, and medical specialists using continuous drug therapy and multiple surgeries, I became a medical disaster by the time I was 45. At one time or another, I suffered all of these symptoms:

Overweight
Unhealthy nails, hair, and skin
Chronic fatigue
Pain in every joint; weak, painful muscles
Severe constipation
Backaches, headaches, and debilitating neck pain
Cold body and extremities all year
Chronic vaginal yeast infections
Decreased sexual desire
PMS and painful periods
Extreme emotional highs and lows; anxiety attacks
Chronic tension and irritability
Frequent colds that could last months
Kidney pain and one kidney stone
Acute gallbladder attack
Sore, burning mouth; frequent mouth sores
Insomnia
Chest pain; very rapid pulse
Stomach pain and nausea after meals
Poor digestion

Doctors never treated my whole body; they merely treated each symptom with drugs or surgery. Eventually I developed an intolerance to most of the drugs they prescribed. When some of their testing showed what they considered to be normal results, my doctors started thinking of me as a hypochondriac because I still had so many symptoms. They had no explanation for my lack of progress, so they said I was "stressed out", and recommended psychiatric counseling. Years of therapy did not improve my general health at all. The only change was an increase in symptoms from the variety of drugs they prescribed for me.

A friend informed me about another kind of doctor who treated food allergies. Since I'd been told everything that could be done was being done, a new doctor didn't seem necessary; I was tired of the frustration and disappointment every time I sought a new physician. When I finally agreed to see this new doctor, my life changed dramatically!

Fuller Royal, M.D. approached my problems from a different point of view. His concern about the CAUSE of my symptoms was a refreshing change from just treating the symptoms. Dr. Royal concluded my problems to be both food allergies and chemical sensitivities. I was hospitalized in a chemically controlled environment under the care of Joseph Morgan, M.D. After a total water fast, I was tested with food not grown with chemical fertilizer or sprayed with any chemical. In two weeks, I learned more about what was actually CAUSING my many symptoms than my other doctors had determined in 20 years. Some of the symptoms connecting with food and chemical testing were:

Beef made me depressed and tearful
Milk gave me joint pains
Corn made my muscles hurt
Soy made my legs ache
Gluten (found in wheat, oats, rye, barley and buckwheat)
    caused rib, chest and stomach pain
Chemicals in my clothing and environment caused headaches,
    fatigue, depression, irritability, and neck pain.

My medical mismanagement left many scars, but none more difficult to deal with than chemical sensitivities. Since World War II, we have become a chemically oriented society. Locating chemical-free food, natural fiber clothing, natural household furnishings, and non-chemical supplies was not easy or inexpensive. Solving my problems quickly was critical; my family was often shocked, frustrated, and angry at how complicated our lives had become.

I was angry at the medical profession for the way they treated me, and resented the loss of enjoyable years and aggravation to my family. The final realization that I was responsible for my own health was difficult to accept, after years of believing medical science would cure me. Making daily choices to heal my body and protect my health was a new way of life.

After a year and a half, I was well enough to work in a holistic health clinic, and organized seminars to share the health techniques I'd learned. I took personal growth seminars, and started teaching classes on positive thinking and stress management. I learned there was more to health than improved diet and avoidance of substances that made me ill. I learned health was on all levels of physical, emotional, mental, and spiritual.

[] [] [] [] [] []

HEALTH METAMORPHOSIS is dedicated to assisting you in making choices for your best health interest, now and in the future. Health is simple. . .it is disease that is complicated. If you practice the principles of the basic laws of wellness, your body can take better care of itself.

Your journey to better health could be likened to a walk on a winding trail. It may turn gradually or have some sharp curves. It may stray occasionally from the main course. With a challenging stream to cross, you may have to control your fear as you balance across a fallen log. You may need to stop and rest. You may wonder how you can go on, but when at last you reach the beautiful view from the summit, you realize it was well worth it.

I want my story to give you new hope. If you are one of the many people who has struggled vainly with modern medicine, you need this book desperately. Application of the information in the next five chapters can perform miracles. I no longer am willing to blindly follow medical recommendations that only treat the symptoms in chronic illness. I would however, seek medical evaluation if following the EIGHT LAWS OF WELLNESS did not produce positive results in a few weeks. Our health care program would benefit greatly by everyone working together with the best of both preventive medicine and modern medicine.

Right now is the perfect time for you to start on your path to metamorphosis! As you consider each new idea, remember you are not going through this alone. Let's turn the page together. . .

CHAPTER 1

POSITIVE THINKING IS POSSIBILITY THINKING

Sometimes life IS rough. Positive thinking does not guarantee you anything; however, negative thinking GUARANTEES it will be harder to deal with your problems. Positive thinking is POSSIBILITY THINKING . . .and that comes from the loving acceptance of yourself. With positive thinking you are OPEN to the options that can make a difference, because you WANT TO ENJOY LIFE. That can be hard. . .or. . .it can be easy. It's your choice!

This poem from *HOW TO SURVIVE THE LOSS OF A LOVE* by Colgrove, Bloomfield, and McWilliams is ALIVE with positive imagery:

> **The world is good.**
> **I feel whole and directed.**
> **Touch my Joy with me.**
> **I cannot keep**
> **my smiles**
> **in single file.**

THE GREATEST CAUSE OF ILLNESS IS NEGATIVE EMOTIONS. You probably believe that continuous stress caused your negative emotions, and there's not much you can do about that because you can't get rid of your stress. You may not be able to take the negative events out of your life, but you can learn to control your ATTITUDE towards them. This quote about attitude is from an unknown source:

> *The longer I live, the more I realize the impact of attitude on life. Attitude, to me, is more important than facts. It is more important than the past, than education, than money, than circumstances, than failures, than successes, than what other people think or say or do. It will make or break a company, a church, a home. The remarkable thing is, we have a choice every day regarding the attitude we embrace for that day. We cannot change the inevitable. The only thing we can do is play the one string we have, and that is our*

How to Survive the Loss of a Love—Colgrove, Bloomfield, and McWilliams (Prelude Press). Reprinted by permission of Prelude Press.

attitude. I am convinced life is 10 percent what happens to me, and 90 percent how I react to it. An so it is with you; we are in charge of our attitudes.

How you think and feel is based a lot on your self-esteem, and affects everything you do. . .every relationship, every task, every choice, every second of your day! The character you develop is from your attitude about your lifetime of trials, errors, and daily struggles that bring out the best in you. . .and CHARACTER BUILDS SELF-ESTEEM.

The will to self-love is the deepest of all desires. You are involved with the greatest adventure of your life. . .to improve your self-esteem, to create more meaning in your life and in the lives of others. Creating a better self-image does not create new abilities, it releases the ones you already have.

> *"LIFE'S GREATEST ACHIEVEMENT IS THE CONTINUAL REMAKING OF YOURSELF SO THAT AT LAST YOU KNOW HOW TO LIVE."* - Norman Vincent Peale

ENTHUSIASM FOR LIFE IS THE MOST IMPORTANT PREDICTOR OF WELLNESS. It is impossible to attain good health without a positive attitude towards life. This is why POSITIVE THINKING is the first chapter of this book. The best diet and exercise program in the world will not provide the health you expect if you don't approach each day and each task with enthusiasm.

> *"FINISH EVERY DAY AND BE DONE WITH IT. YOU HAVE DONE WHAT YOU COULD. SOME BLUNDERS AND ABSURDITIES NO DOUBT CREPT IN; FORGET THEM AS SOON AS YOU CAN. TOMORROW IS A NEW DAY; BEGIN IT WELL AND SERENELY. THIS DAY IS ALL THAT IS GOOD AND FAIR. IT IS TOO DEAR, WITH ITS HOPES AND INVITATIONS, TO WASTE A MOMENT ON THE YESTERDAYS."* - Ralph Waldo Emerson

Most people, at one time or another, transfer their energy in negative directions. . .towards conflict, stagnation, and isolation. To be healthy, you must learn to channel your energy in a direction that will build health. Wisdom is knowing what to do next! Wisdom lies in the ability to forgive ourselves and others of human failings; and when we tumble, pick ourselves up and learn from the experience. Today you are learning to do it better tomorrow. That's what life is all about. . .to become stronger (not weaker) from your experiences.

[] [] [] [] [] []

It all starts with positive energy. That increases your ENTHUSIASM so you want to participate in life, not just observe it. If you dread Saturday night, Sundays are no fun, and holidays are even worse, you need to take a good look at YOURSELF. A person who CHOOSES to be lonely any day can also CHOOSE not to. . .any day! Don't allow television to fill all your time. It should be used for information or relaxation, but not for a way to escape from life. GET INTO ACTION:

* **Take personal development seminars or lectures, read personal growth books, or listen to personal growth tapes.** They assist in bringing out the giant that's inside you.

* **Take an adult education class or other educational opportunity** through a university, community college, or city parks department (I took flower identification, bird watching, and animal tracking classes to enrich my hikes). The effort will expand your horizons, and reward you both in learning and social enjoyment. TO SEARCH IS TO NEVER EXPERIENCE BOREDOM!

* **Connect with your creator** and let the light that shines within provide the enthusiasm that will be your driving force.

   "I AM POSITIVELY ADDICTED TO GIVING PEOPLE HOPE."   - Robert H. Schuller

* **Experience creativity** by DOING what you want to do, not just thinking about it. The only thing that stops the creative person inside you is your negative subconscious (that you put there).

> *A friend admired my oil paintings and said she'd always wanted to paint, but denied her ability. When I finally persuaded her to paint with me, she completed a beautiful mountain scene. She displays her work with pride, and enjoys telling people she can paint.*

All the poems I've written in my life have been at the height of feeling good about myself. Poetry is an effective balancing mechanism because it is both left brain logical, and right brain creative. Thus, it can balance the cerebral hemispheres and reduce tension.

> *"INSTEAD OF ONE ASPIRIN, TAKE TWO POEMS."*
> *- psychiatrist Dr. Jack Leedy,*
> *when his patients have trouble sleeping.*

* **Get involved in fun activities** because life does not always have to be a struggle. Play may be the most vital thing you do, because it will renew you. If you can't enjoy a good time, and you feel like a victim, you may be coming from the belief system that you can't be happy, and life is hard. Through your negative thoughts and choices you will make sure it stays that way, because it confirms your belief system.

When you are having fun, you also need to learn the art of relaxation. Unfortunately, many people try to relax at the same pace that they lead the rest of their lives. True relaxation is becoming sensitive to one's basic needs for self-awareness and thoughtful reflection. Many people are so pressure oriented they do not take time to satisfy their own basic needs. That is an almost guaranteed program for illness. Our production oriented society is so task directed that even vacations become whirlwind projects.

> *"REST IS ACTION WITHOUT FRICTION."*
> - Robert H. Schuller

Remember RELAXATION and not achievement is your main goal. Two important rules in deciding what activity to pick are:

1. Do not be afraid to try something new and different.
2. Choose the activity YOU enjoy, not always what other people want you to do.

* **Laughing** gives the body a mini-workout, as it involves virtually every major body system. For millions of people life is like a toothache with no money to see a dentist. They finally give up and accept the pain with all the elements of being a victim. They struggle for survival using negative manipulation, and are shocked when life gets worse. They lose a valuable link to survival. . .humor!

[] [] [] [] [] []

HOW TO RESOLVE A PROBLEM

We can't laugh all day if there are real problems. To resolve a problem, you need a plan. Always remember that ACTION is the antidote for worry. Have a separate piece of paper for each problem, and answer the following questions **on each problem.** Then prioritize them in order of urgency, and decide on a place to start!

- **WHAT IS THE REAL PROBLEM?**
Many people worry before they get all the facts. Deal only with the facts! A situation handled with all the facts correct, could keep a problem from getting out of hand.

- **WHAT IS THE CAUSE OF THE PROBLEM?**
This should give you some hints on how to deal with it. Remember to assume responsibility for any part you play in the problem.

- **WHAT ARE ALL THE POSSIBLE SOLUTIONS?**
No one can know all the uncertainties, but you can give an educated guess to the solutions based on the known facts. This is the time to think, and not be emotional. Future

"what-ifs" and past "if-onlys" can only drive you crazy with speculation. It keeps you in a negative attitude that prevents you from forming a GAME PLAN to resolve the issue.

- PICK A POSSIBLE SOLUTION AND ACT ON IT! WORRY IS DEFINITELY NOT ACTION! Worry is a negative thought that wastes energy...and that can prevent you from solving the problem. One of the biggest causes of chronic worry is low self-esteem.

However, when you worry with a positive mental attitude, it can be to your advantage, and lead to solutions.

DEAL WITH THE FACTS
ACT ON THE FACTS
DO THE BEST YOU CAN TODAY...BECAUSE TODAY IS THE TOMORROW YOU WORRIED ABOUT YESTERDAY!

"WE SHALL HAVE NO BETTER CONDITIONS IN THE FUTURE IF WE ARE SATISFIED WITH ALL THOSE WHICH WE HAVE AT PRESENT."
— Thomas Edison

[] [] [] [] [] []

Reorganize priorities because you deserve a part of each day for yourself. If you're swamped with tasks you don't feel like doing, or responsibilities not of your own choosing, perhaps it's time to reorganize your priorities. If you believe your life is not under your control, you should examine your self-esteem.

Your self-esteem may not always be from conscious thoughts, but may be from your subconscious. Your subconscious is the source of information for your conscious mind, and stores all the beliefs you have collected over your lifetime. Many of those beliefs are not who you really are, but are based on your interpretation of how others see you. So, your subconscious is developed both from WHAT OTHERS SAY TO YOU, and WHAT YOU SAY TO YOURSELF. If those beliefs are experienced often enough, you'll become the person you believe others think you are.

Three examples of how negative childhood programming from others, and your own negative thinking can mold your adult thinking are:

- A child may be scolded continually by the mother for being slow. The mother may be tense and constantly overextended, and the child may not be unusually slow at all. However, the child will grow up thinking he/she is slow because the mother firmly implanted the thought. Symptoms like low productivity, indecision, habitual tardiness and inability to speed up the pace when needed may appear as the child grows.

- Comparison with a bright sibling may lead to feeling intellectually inferior. In high school, I was frequently referred to as "Lawrence's sister." Since I did not think I could compete with my brother's intelligence, I decided to play a lighthearted clown role to avoid comparison. Blocking my intellectual awareness followed me for years. I performed well, but my belief system prevented me from acknowledging my accomplishments. It took years of working on self-esteem to overcome this inhibiting behavior.

- Someone who felt unloved as a child might be too involved in the PROCESS of looking for love to recognize love if it occurred. He/she might also get involved in a problem relationship because of the belief they do not deserve better. A person who did not feel special as a child, or felt unloved, may wonder who would care. Daily negative choices will set him/her up to continue the negative belief that *I can't be happy and life is hard.*

You also have a creative subconscious that is the REAL you! But creativity can only be developed with positive thoughts; you cannot be creative with negative energy. You can't always control what others say to you, but YOU CAN ALWAYS CONTROL WHAT YOU SAY TO YOURSELF! The more POSITIVE you think, the less likely you will continue to be influenced by your interpretation of negative childhood experiences. You are now free to make choices that will develop the creative YOU.

> *Jess Lair in his book I AIN'T MUCH BABY, BUT I'M ALL I'VE GOT, feels the best psychology he has found in 45 years of research is:* "YOU CAN SOLVE ALL YOUR PROBLEMS THAT CAN BE SOLVED BY GOING IN SEARCH OF THE MAGNIFICENT 'YOU', AND AN ADDED REWARD FOR THAT IS THE ACCEPTANCE OF OTHERS WHICH FREES THEM TO SEARCH FOR THEMSELVES, TOO."

[] [] [] [] [] []

All personality is not hereditary; much is a learned behavior. As children, we constantly want to please, and we quickly learn what behaviors are expected from us. We often suppress our own personality if it conflicts with what we think others want us to be. The result is an internal tug-of-war that can continue for life. Many adults with suppressed personalities had at least one very dominant parent.

In a single parent home, a child may try even harder to please the remaining parent. If the parent has a controlling personality, and takes charge too often, the child may not develop decision-making normally. As an adult, he/she may have problems with productivity, creativity, and self-image. This usually surfaces as a real problem about mid-life when that adult realizes the need to feel in charge of his/her life. It's one reason some people make drastic changes during this period of their lives.

We often marry, or develop partnerships to strengthen our own weaknesses. Instead of two people being individuals, they combine to make up one personality. This process is called SYMBIOSIS, and is another cause of mid-life crisis. For mental and emotional health, a person needs full development of the personality's three aspects: the child state (ability to have fun), the parent state (ability to take care of oneself), and the adult state (intellectual development). One reason we have negative thoughts about ourselves is because we see our own weaknesses. We all want to feel confident, responsible, intelligent, and willing to have fun; we all want to be in charge of our child, parent and adult states.

In the positive use of symbiosis, neither consenting person is harmed; and the association is beneficial to both. What happens too often, is the basic human need to feel like a WHOLE, CAPABLE PERSON is not being satisfied for one of the participants. This now unsatisfied basic need irritates that person into resenting the association. Now the union is not beneficial, and marital or partnership problems develop. For example, a man with a poor child state marries a vivacious girl who in mid-life decides to develop a more serious intellectual side. The man may not appreciate the wife's new image, if he is still lacking a child state.

Many people simply don't know how to have fun; they have an undeveloped child state. Growing up with a struggling single parent, financial hardship, or family disaster can damage one's child state. Life was hard for the child. As an adult, his/her belief confirms that life is hard, by being unwilling to have fun. They become couch-potatoes, victims, introverts, or "bah humbug" year round.

[] [] [] [] [] []

Creativity can be one of the most enjoyable ways to put fun in a person's life. It can make a career stimulating, raising children more fun, and provide productive ways of filling time. It is a sad waste when a person's natural ability to be creative is blocked by negative subconscious beliefs. If your subconscious holds doubts about your intelligence, talent, or leadership qualities, you may go through life holding back, and have one disappointment after another.

You can decide today how you want to see yourself, and how you wish others to see you. To change your image, you need to reprogram your subconscious, and let that wonderful unblocked creativity take over. You can do this by using the following techniques:

* **Deep relaxation tapes** - these are available through some health food stores, some bookstores, and health magazines.

* **Counseling** - be careful! Find a counselor who deals with the issues in a positive, forward energy, and doesn't keep you locked in the past.

* **Neurolinguistic Programming (NLP)** - the technique assists you in communicating with your subconscious, and changing whatever is needed to gain control over your life. It also assists you in communicating with others. Check a bookstore for books available to teach yourself the techniques.

* **Affirmations** - these are positive thoughts you choose to put in your conscious mind. If you repeat the affirmation often enough, the information will be stored in your subconscious, and you will begin to believe it is true.

You become what you think you are. If you think you are successful, then you become successful. If you think you are stupid, or slow, then you become stupid or slow. The words you use to describe yourself are very powerful. . .SO STOP THE STINKING THINKING! You either program yourself, or are influenced by other people's thoughts or words. Your mind controls your actions, emotions, and attitudes, based on the information it receives. So, if you keep telling your mind you can't do anything right, is it surprising that you'll find yourself doing everything wrong? Use positive words to change bad habits, establish new ones, and develop new patterns of behavior. Affirmations greatly assist a person with an intense determination to change. Try these techniques:

- **Personalize the affirmation** by saying, "I, (name), am successful."

- **Acknowledge other people have conditioned you.** Look into a mirror and say, "You, (name), are successful." Eye to eye contact in the mirror directs the affirmation to you. Whenever possible, use your mirror.

- **State your affirmations in the present tense,** as though you've already achieved your goal. For example, never say, "I plan to become successful." This gives you an excuse for not being successful NOW. Instead say, "I AM successful!" Remember, you are developing a **POSITIVE BELIEF SYSTEM** that will help you make choices to confirm your new beliefs.

- **State your affirmations in the positive form.** Instead of saying, "I do not want to smoke," say, "I, (name), make healthy choices for my well being."

- **Repeat your affirmation throughout the day.** Your brain will eventually get the message, and will believe anything you tell it often enough. State your affirmations when you first get up, as often as possible throughout the day, and the last thing before retiring.

> *One day I was stating my "successful" affirmation while waiting for a red light to change. It reminded me to call a contact I'd known about for several months. I called as soon as I got home, and the effort resulted in a professional opportunity, plus a radio and a television interview.* ***POSITIVE AFFIRMATIONS HELP KEEP YOU ACTION-ORIENTED!***

- **Be firm and don't stop just because you don't believe it yet.** You may laugh when you look in the mirror and say, "I, (name), am beautiful," but that won't prevent exciting changes from occurring if you keep saying it. You'll become motivated to make those changes, and you'll learn to see yourself in a different way. You'll see beauty as more than surface appearance; and may also decide to make changes that could improve the way you look to yourself and others.

Affirmations can be acting rather than verbal. If you wake up some morning feeling depressed or irritable, force yourself to be pleasant to the first person you see. You'll find your whole attitude changing. You can choose to stay depressed or irritable, BUT WHAT A WASTE OF ENERGY THAT IS!!!

[] [] [] [] [] []

Have you ever listened carefully to someone with a negative attitude? Try it sometime, and recall the words or phrases they use most often. You'll hear a lot of words like:

I want to, but	perhaps	so-so
I hope so	maybe	I don't know
I wish I could	later	I can't help it
I plan to someday	I'll try	possibly

These negative people exhaust their energy. "I am trying" means nothing. You either ARE, or you ARE NOT making your life work for you. Change your vocabulary, and imagine what your day could be like. The reward for hanging on to negative words is AVOIDANCE; you don't have to deal with challenge. You start the day with all your "comfort zones," and end the day with lost opportunities to learn and enjoy life. Replace negative words with positive words like:

I will	yes	I would love to
I do	now	that's exciting
I can	definitely	I care
let's go	I'll help	certainly

You may believe negative things about yourself, and you will act accordingly to confirm these negative beliefs. . .TIME AND TIME AGAIN! If you can admit your own negative thoughts, you can now CONSCIOUSLY choose to change your attitude.

Shyness is a widespread psychological problem of Americans today. Picture yourself as you would like to be. . .then practice positive affirmations. You must first communicate with yourself before you will successfully venture out and be comfortable with others.

THE THREE WAYS TO REPROGRAM THE SUBCONSCIOUS ARE:

- **POSITIVE AFFIRMATIONS** - I AM SOMETHING, AND I WILL MAKE THE MOST OF THAT SOMETHING, is a good positive affirmation.

- **WILL AND DETERMINATION** - You simply have had enough of the way your life has been going, and you WILL make it better!!!

- USE THE WORD "OR" TO CHANGE NEGATIVE WORDS OR THOUGHTS TO POSITIVE WORDS OR THOUGHTS - as soon as you say or think, "I'll never learn that", follow it immediately with, "Or, I will". Listen to your own words or thoughts. You may be surprised how often you sabotage your day.

[] [] [] [] [] []

No one wants to be sick or unmotivated; there has to be some kind of a *pay-off* for a person to hang on to illness. People want to be healthy and successful. . .unless, of course, they don't. If this is the case, something in the negative subconscious is getting satisfied. I'll qualify this by saying continuous stress may have created minor symptoms at first, but, treating only the symptoms without getting to the cause of the problems can lead to more stress, and more symptoms. Then, poor diet choices, nutritional deficiencies, allergies, chemical sensitivities, hiding out in addictive habits, taking unnecessary drugs with multiple side effects, or not living by laws that promote health can make simple symptoms into out-of-control symptoms. The person may now be sick on all levels - physical, emotional and mental. HOW IT ALL GOT STARTED IS LOST IN THE CRISIS.

A person with negative subconscious programs will usually make a lot of wrong health choices. Their deteriorating health keeps them in the VICTIM state, and they actually become "comfortable in their discomfort". For them, the *pay-off* is **CONFIRMING** that "I can't be happy, and life is hard".

This poem from *HOW TO SURVIVE THE LOSS OF A LOVE* may be the way you've felt at some time:

> I sat evaluating
> myself.
> I decided
> to lie down.

WHY DO PEOPLE WHO TRULY BELIEVE THEY'D LIKE TO BE HEALTHY CONTINUE TO EXPERIENCE POOR HEALTH? Here are just a few examples of pay-offs:

- **TO AVOID INTIMACY** - Using the old saying, "Not now, I've got a headache", has been expanded to include backache, stomachache, muscle pain or any other body symptom. It works every time, because our society is very "symptom" oriented. Poor health is used successfully to keep people away.

- **GETTING THE JOB YOU WANT** - Poor health can get you changed from a job you don't like to one you prefer. You may keep a backache until you get the sit-down job you wanted. You may stay unemployed or plagued with bad breaks, because that confirms your belief that you are not capable of success.

- **TO AVOID RESPONSIBILITY** - If you're afraid of competing or assuming responsibility, you may become introverted. People are not born shy. They get that way because there is a pay-off confirming a belief that they are weak and unimportant.

☐ ☐ ☐ ☐ ☐ ☐

MINDTRAPS KEEP YOU LOCKED IN THE PAST

Your state of mind has much to do with your control over life. The way you respond to any situation is your reaction based on the beliefs in your subconscious mind. This reaction, called a **MINDTRAP**, is the way you deal with suppressed fear and insecurity. Mindtraps keep you locked in suppressed trauma or negative childhood teachings. Accept the past for the good and the bad in it. . .then go on with your life. You cannot undo the past, but you can accept it and learn from past experiences to make you stronger. **YOU** are now in charge of the present and the future. Acknowledging a mindtrap is a start to understanding what you are suppressing. Mindtraps prevent you from coping with:

- **THE PRESENT** - Living in the past is easier than challenging the present, and you never have to develop your potential.

- **SUPPRESSED TRAUMA** - You stay locked in, and haunted by past negative experiences.

- **NEGATIVE CHILDHOOD TEACHINGS** - You do not give yourself credit for being in control of your life now.

SOME EXAMPLES OF MINDTRAPS ARE:

- **GUILT** - You're feeling guilty about everything. "I'm sure I'm the one to blame." "I'm the one who causes all the trouble." You apologize constantly. Suppressed trauma like this can occur from guilt over injuring a loved one, parent's divorce, or other family crisis you caused. . .or think you caused.

- **MISTRUST** - You don't trust love, friendship, job security, or anything else. Childhood abuse, physical or emotional neglect, or abandonment can result in serious mistrust.

- **CONFUSION** - In childhood you may have felt incompetent, so living in chaos keeps people from giving you responsibility.

- **DEFENSIVENESS** - Physical or verbal harassment in childhood produces this mindtrap.

- **SHAME** - This mindtrap can result from poor handling by adults of childhood events, like stealing or sexual issues.

- **RATIONALIZATION** - This excuses one's conscious act without realizing the real subconscious motive. "It's okay to lie if it helps you get ahead." You do what is needed, and may not consciously acknowledge the driving force from the past.

There are many mindtraps like regret, humiliation, emptiness, resentment, resignation, explanation, self-righteousness, and others. Remember, for better or for worse, the past was part of your life. Accept it; now deal with the present and the future. . .you don't have to live in a world of mindtraps.

[] [] [] [] [] []

BOTH BEHAVIOR AND FEELINGS COME FROM YOUR BELIEFS. IF YOU DON'T LIKE THE WAY YOUR LIFE IS GOING , ASK YOURSELF:

- **IS THERE A GOOD REASON FOR MY BELIEF?** If so, are you letting a past experience you had no control over affect today, which you DO have control over?

    A baby circus elephant is restrained with a well secured chain, and struggles but cannot get free. As he grows, the secured chain is bigger and stronger. After a while, believing he cannot get loose, he stops struggling. A huge elephant in the circus is restrained with only a small peg in the ground. Many adults behave like the circus elephant, restrained in thought and action all their lives based on a belief system.

- **COULD I BE MISTAKEN IN MY BELIEF?** Could your interpretation of the situation be changed with more understanding, compassion, or change in attitude?

- **EVEN IF MY BELIEF IS TRUE, SHOULD I CONTINUE LETTING IT INFLUENCE MY LIFE?**

    "I'M NOT FREE UNTIL I BELIEVE IN ME."
    — Robert H. Schuller

- **DO I REALLY HAVE A COMMITMENT TO IMPROVE THE QUALITY OF MY LIFE?** IF NOT...WHY WOULD I WANT TO LIVE EACH DAY THE SAME AS BEFORE?

[] [] [] [] [] []

WAYS TO ENHANCE YOUR POTENTIAL

Everyone has the power within himself/herself to produce a giant. Most people only use a fraction of their capabilities. To create a better self-image does not create NEW abilities...it RELEASES the ones you already have! To enhance your potential:

1. **PARTICIPATE in life 100 percent rather than living as an observer...GET ACTIVE!** Procrastination is the art of keeping up with yesterday. It's alright to be lazy occasionally. This may sound like a paradox, but a person works best who

can relax enough to assimilate daily experiences, renew their energy and take time to plan. The word is BALANCE.

> *"THERE ARE NO RULES HERE; WE'RE TRYING TO GET SOMETHING DONE."* - Thomas Edison

2. **BE HONEST with yourself and others,** if you expect others to be honest with you. If you tell the truth you don't have to remember anything.

3. **TRUST your own judgment.** Make a list of your best qualities, and don't be afraid to pat yourself on the back!

4. **ACCEPT other points of view.** Unless you listen to what someone else says, all you can base your opinion on is what you THINK you know.

5. **COMMUNICATE with people.** Observe people's response to how you speak to them. Be clear and concise so people don't just hear what you say, but understand what you mean. The following two statements, "You have a face that could stop a clock," and "When I look at you time stands still," have the same meaning, but can be interpreted very differently.

6. **SUPPORT others to win in life;** everyone loves a supporter. Share your experiences; be a good listener. Act as if other people are important.

> *"I CAN GO TWO WEEKS WITH ONE COMPLIMENT FROM A FRIEND."* - Mark Twain

To handle yourself, use your head; to handle others, use your heart.

> *"BE SOMEONE FOR SOMEBODY."*
> - Mother Teresa

7. **DO NOT LIVE IN DAILY JUDGMENT of others.** You don't know all the facts about another person's life, so you cannot **accurately** assess how their experiences have affected

them. Everyone does the best they can at any given time. Just like you, they may have had many experiences that left scars. Not everyone has the opportunity to learn what makes them think, feel, or act the way they do...so...THEY DO THE BEST THEY CAN DO AT THE TIME! Don't try to change anyone but yourself! You will like, or understand almost everyone you meet better, after you get to know them.

8. **FORGIVE who you are angry at;** they did the best they could do at the time. Then forgive yourself for reacting. Understand that nobody is perfect, including you. Don't be so hard on yourself in a learning situation. Everyone is ignorant...only on different subjects. It is necessary to recognize your shortcomings, but disastrous to hate yourself for them.

9. **TOUCH is an exchange of "energy",** and that is what makes the world go round. "Reach out and touch someone" is more than a telephone commercial. A touch is worth a thousand words because it means what life is all about...caring. Touchers are usually less afraid, less tense, and less suspicious of others. Non-touchers tend to be more internal, unstable, apprehensive, and usually have low self-esteem.

10. **BE YOURSELF;** dump phony images. Admit you are flawed, but you are becoming...!

    "KNOW YOURSELF! DON'T ACCEPT YOUR DOG'S ADMIRATION AS CONCLUSIVE EVIDENCE THAT YOU ARE WONDERFUL."   - Ann Landers

11. **BE FLEXIBLE** and willing to try something else if what you want out of life is not happening. Just because it is a well-worn path, does not mean it is the right one. Commit yourself to your belief system, if it works for you; be willing to change if it does not.

    "THIS TIME, LIKE ALL OTHER TIMES, IS A VERY GOOD ONE, IF WE BUT KNEW WHAT TO DO WITH IT."   - Ralph Waldo Emerson

12. **LOVE YOURSELF.** If you don't love yourself, why should anyone else love you? YOU ARE GREAT. . .AND GETTING BETTER! Give yourself credit for each small success. With self-confidence comes leadership. . .and with leadership comes charisma. CHARISMA IS JUST AN ATTITUDE OF CONFIDENCE!

13. **HAVE FUN!** Learn to live life in the experiential sensory groups: visual (sight), auditory (hearing), kinesthetic (feeling), gustatory (taste), and olfactory (smell). Tuning out any one diminishes your awareness. In our society, sight is often tuned out; your home may not be what you want, or you don't enjoy your personal appearance. A noisy neighborhood, job, or noisy children, may make you tune out hearing. Avoidance of intimacy or traumatic emotional crisis can tune out feeling. Blocking sensory experiences diminishes your awareness, and that can reduce opportunities that could add pleasure to your life.

    Think of going to the mountains, **SEEING** the spectacular view, **HEARING** the wind and water, **SMELLING** the woods aroma, **FEELING** a soft velvet flower, and **TASTING** your delicious lunch. That sort of breathtakingly complete sensory experience is what having fun, and enjoying life is all about.

    We should not have to look back on the "carefree days of childhood" as though they are completely gone. Some adults never allow themselves that sort of non-goal directed behavior; they're always trying to accomplish something. It's not important what you play. . .IT'S JUST IMPORTANT THAT YOU PLAY! Growing up for some people is not fun. What they don't realize is that if they had not lost the ability to play along the way, life might have been easier. Perhaps the single most outstanding characteristic of healthy people is their SENSE OF HUMOR.

14. **LEARN about your behavior** by observing how you respond to situations. If you smoke or eat every time you get tense, the negative addiction will be very hard to break because it not only pacifies the struggle, but actually provides a

pleasurable experience. You substitute the addictive pattern, and accept that it is alright because you enjoy it so much.. Smokers like to smoke...overeater like to eat...drinkers like to drink. This enjoyment prevents you from facing the REASON for the addiction.

Keep promises and be reliable; be on time for appointments. If this is a problem, you need to look for a mindtrap, or a pay-off.

15. **BE ACCOUNTABLE for what you do.** The greatest fault is to be conscious of none.

16. **COMMIT to winning in life.** This doesn't necessarily imply financial or career success; winning in life means being the best in whatever is most important to you.

> **IF YOU WANT TO DO IT...DO IT!**
> **IF YOU WANT TO LEARN IT...LEARN IT!**
> **ONLY YOU CAN STOP YOUR CREATIVITY**
> **WHICH IS ALREADY THERE!**

> *"THE MOST GLORIOUS MOMENTS IN YOUR LIFE ARE NOT THE SO-CALLED DAYS OF SUCCESS, BUT RATHER THOSE DAYS WHEN OUT OF DEJECTION AND DESPAIR, YOU FEEL RISE IN YOU A CHALLENGE TO LIFE, AND THE PROMISE OF FUTURE ACCOMPLISHMENTS."*
> — Gustave Flaubert

The three C's - commitment, control, and challenge are the ingredients of "hardiness." Hardy people face change with confidence; less hardy people feel threatened. Hardy people stay healthier, even with a strong family history of disease, than people who cannot cope.

> *Sir Ernest Shackleton ran this ad in a London paper for an Antarctic expedition:* MEN WANTED FOR HAZARDOUS JOURNEY, SMALL WAGES, BITTER COLD, LONG MONTHS OF COMPLETE DARKNESS, CONSTANT DANGER, SAFE RETURN DOUBTFUL.

*HONOR AND RECOGNITION IN CASE OF SUCCESS."
When all returned alive, he wrote: "WE PIERCED THE
VENEER OF OUTSIDE THINGS, AND REACHED THE
NAKED SOUL OF MAN."*

How can you learn to be hardy? **By viewing daily stressors in ways that produce MINIMAL stress response.** A person of conviction must choose one side of the road or the other. . . not the middle of the road. . .or on the fence! Few people today reach the depth of human satisfaction that is the ultimate of hardiness. In our soft, modern ways we have forgotten how to be tough enough to reach our naked soul. Too often we:

- play it safe
- aim for the sure thing
- want life to be easy
- seldom stretch ourselves

17. **BE RECEPTIVE to new ideas.** New ideas can make you fearful, but fear is a limiting belief that keeps you from what you want. Learn more about what you fear; you'll reduce or eliminate the fear. Don't be afraid of a challenge. What you don't know, you can always learn.

    Change is good, but to enjoy life to the fullest, remember balance. We need both paved highways, and trails through quiet woods. We need television, but also time to see flying geese in the fall.

18. **CELEBRATE LIFE each day.** Even with daily problems and challenges, you should enjoy the experience of living. Your Creator has a plan for you. You are on earth for two reasons:

    - to learn and grow
    - to be in service to humankind

*"I WAS RICH, IF NOT IN MONEY, IN SUNNY HOURS
AND SUMMER DAYS."*   - Henry David Thoreau

I wrote a poem about enjoying life:

*The day begins
the dawn arrives
Down around my face supplies my needs.
Sunbeams invite me
Song birds delight me
Oh day, JOYFUL DAY.*

*Another day the clouds appear
The rain drowns out the birds I hear.
No matter,
I still have the sun in me.
Oh day, JOYFUL DAY!*

❑ ❑ ❑ ❑ ❑ ❑

In the movie about Eleanor Roosevelt, she said, **"FEAR IS AN ILLUSION. IF YOU PUT THE SAME ENERGY IN CONFIDENCE, THE MOST WONDERFUL THINGS HAPPEN."** Eleanor Roosevelt's life was filled with accomplishments, because she had a positive attitude. If you approach every day, every task, and every goal with the same enthusiasm, you too can accomplish "wonderful things". . . CHALLENGE YOURSELF!

A personal fear was challenged by signing up for a two-day raft trip without the support of my husband. Beneath my fascination with rafting was a genuine fear of the water. The orientation included a whitewater movie that left me sinking into my chair. By the end of the film I left fingernail marks on the man next to me; he was so scared he didn't feel anything.

We were told to dress in light layers, but positive I'd end up in the cold water, I wore long underwear and warm ski clothes. I looked pretty strange crawling into the boat nest to people in bathing suits. The black electric tape securing my glasses was disturbing to me, since a class on my best colors suggested black was not my color.

The adventure ran me through the whole gamut of emotions from abject terror to pride. Emotions by the end of the day were both excitement and relief; I'd actually survived. By the end of the second day (in my bathing suit), fulfillment was overwhelming. Respect for the river had replaced fear. Satisfaction had replaced wishful thinking. I'd challenged more than the river; I'd challenged myself.

By confronting one fear, it would be easier to confront others. I used to think I had to have someone with me for support. I had someone this time. . .myself! In the future, my positive energy will be reinforced by new confidence. Discovering the joys of living with a beginner's mind will no longer be a problem.

I'm not suggesting that you challenge every fear you have. I do not choose to skydive or climb rocks, so those fears do not contain negative energy. Any situation you'd like to participate in, but are afraid to, contains negative energy. Put that energy into confidence and learn what you need to learn; the most wonderful things will happen!

[] [] [] [] [] []

Experience, good or bad, is what you learn from, or what you do with what happens to you. The source of experience is what is happening WITHIN you, not the actual event. No event or series of events should control what a person becomes. That should be under his/her control. . . thus, experience results from one's handling of life's joys, triumphs, sorrows, and defeats.

The question is not, "ARE YOU PERFECT?". . .but, "ARE YOU LEARNING FROM YOUR MISTAKES?!"

In his senior year in high school, my youngest son's baseball team was hoping to be in the championship series, when they lost an early game in the third extra inning. Frustrated, my son slammed his fist towards the side of the dugout, but hit the drainpipe instead and broke his hand. He could have gone into depression, or played on the sympathy of this teammates and family, but he chose differently. He accepted the situation with maturity and accountability. *He spent the rest of the season in a cast, but was such a team booster he got the* Most Inspirational Player *award, and a $500 college scholarship for* Best All-Around Team Member.

The experience, for him, was not the broken hand; it was the opportunity to accept a difficult situation (which was the outcome of his own actions), and make it a positive experience. He learned some valuable character traits can be built out of adversity.

[] [] [] [] [] []

If you don't like the way you are, YOU HAVE THE POWER TO CHANGE, but you shouldn't believe you have the right to change others. Learn to enjoy the people around you for who they are. You have to deal with many different people in life; you will only frustrate yourself if you can't accept each one for their own uniqueness. Possibility thinking is different for everyone.

What makes people act the way they do? Why do they act differently than you? We all belong, in one way or another, to different personality groups. The four basic groups are: ANALYST, SUPPORTER, CONTROLLER, and PROMOTER. You may have traits in all four groups, or be strong in three, have a combination of two, or be intense in one. There is a positive and a negative side to each personality, and you will experience each at one time or another. Don't apologize because you clearly belong to any one group. . .the truth is:

> **You are not *inferior*.**
> **You are not *superior*.**
> **You are simply *you*.**

TO FIND YOUR DOMINANT PERSONALITY GROUP ASK IF:

MOST OF THE TIME do you prefer to be in charge, or do you prefer someone else to be in charge?
MOST OF THE TIME are you formal in the precision of your work or do you have a more relaxed attitude about details?

If you are NOT DOMINANT and FORMAL most of the time, you are an analyst.
If you are NOT DOMINANT and INFORMAL most of the time, you are a supporter.
If you are DOMINANT and FORMAL most of the time, you are a controller.
If you are DOMINANT and INFORMAL most of the time, you are a promoter.

You'll enjoy your family, your co-workers, your friends, and even yourself more if you stretch out of your own personality quadrant into the quadrant of other people. Appreciate people for who THEY are. Share your talents, but don't force your beliefs on others. THERE ARE LESSONS TO BE LEARNED BY OBSERVING, RATHER THAN DOMINATING! The one thing you should know for sure, is that there is an awful lot you do not know...stretch yourself!

BASIC PERSONALITY GROUPS

ANALYST - NOT DOMINANT AND FORMAL

POSITIVE TRAITS	NEGATIVE TRAITS
Industrious	Critical/Picky
Persistent	Indecisive
Serious/Sensible	Resistant
Exacting/Detailed	Stuffy/Moralistic
Orderly/Logical	Can overdo details
Data gathering	Reluctant initiative
Enjoys learning	Shies away from emotion

SUPPORTER - NOT DOMINANT AND INFORMAL

POSITIVE TRAITS	NEGATIVE TRAITS
Pliable/Supportive	Can move slowly/Unsure
Enjoys people/Family oriented	Communicates poorly
Willing/Agreeable	Needs timetable
Quick to accept	Can be wishy-washy
Conforming	Reluctant to be tough
Respectful	Procrastinates
Dependable	Needs precise information

CONTROLLER - DOMINANT AND FORMAL

POSITIVE TRAITS
Strong-willed/Independent
Practical
Individualized
Businesslike
Decisive/Observant
Efficient/Selective
Maximum potential

NEGATIVE TRAITS
Pushy/Dominating
Brusque/Severe/Harsh
Expects much of others
Demanding
Perfectionist
May be too selective
Speed too important

PROMOTER - DOMINANT AND INFORMAL

POSITIVE TRAITS
Ambitious
Enthusiastic/Lots of hustle
Friendly/Likes people
Communicates
Likes adventure
Stimulating/Dramatic
Likes a challenge

NEGATIVE TRAITS
Manipulative
Undisciplined/Impulsive
Egotistical
Can be sloppy
Can overlook fine points
Overly talkative/Excitable
Impatient

Understanding the personalities of people with whom you associate can be helpful in communicating with them. Some examples are:

- **CHILDREN** - I had an analyst child and a supporter child. If I'd known this at critical times, I could have prevented many problems. Don't compare children; they are beautifully different. Allow children to be themselves and not a forced carbon copy of you.

- **CO-WORKERS** - If you are unable to get along with a particular co-worker, information about his/her personality group can help you better understand how to be flexible in the situation.

- **STAFF** - Office staffing needs to be balanced. Two strong controllers in one area can be destructive. A whole office of strong controllers would be disastrous! A whole office of promoters want time to play. Supporters without leadership won't be able to make positive changes. Analysts will be so busy with details that productivity could be reduced.

- **YOURSELF** - The negative side of your personality shows how you can create problems for yourself. It may also show that you are too dominant in one group. The most balanced personality has some traits in each group.

I know a lady who appeared to be a supporter but was often unhappy and unhealthy. During a seminar she discovered that as a child, she didn't want to grow up to be like her very strong, controlling mother. When she realized that it was possible to be a nice controller, she expanded her talents and assumed the more comfortable role of leadership. Her stress tolerance, and her health improved.

- **RELATIONSHIPS** - There are two combinations that typically tend to have problems. One is analyst/controller. The analyst wants all the data before making a decision, and is very irritating to the decisive controller. The other disastrous combination would be two inflexible controllers. Battle lines are drawn, and the fur flies.

COMBINATIONS THAT WORK WELL TOGETHER:

Two Analysts: They can get along amicably, but an excess of logic and order might make this relationship subdued!

A Supporter and an Analyst, or two Supporters: They make an effective team, but the relationship may lack spark. Supporters give support to any other personality.

A Promoter works well with all four personality groups: They add fun and excitement to the supporter or analyst's life..

Two FLEXIBLE Controllers: They can get along, as long as they allow each other equal time to be in control.

[] [] [] [] [] []

Many people received valuable lessons from their parents that set the stage for maturity. They become stronger from early lessons, and are ready to deal with life's challanges as their life evolves. Other people need to *find their strength* as an adult, because their childhood was filled with stress. *Knowing who you are helps you make the most of **today**.* Today is the most important day in your life. . .yesterday is over, and tomorrow has not come.

"WHAT YOU ARE IS YOUR FOLK'S FAULT. BUT, IF YOU STAY THAT WAY, IT IS YOUR FAULT."
                              - unknown author in freshman psychology class

You are in charge of your life now. You are either thinking in a positive or negative way...THERE IS NO ALMOST-POSITIVE. We can program ourselves for failure by harping self-criticism and victim stories...OR...we can program ourselves for success by TAKING CHARGE OF OUR ENERGY AND DOING SOMETHING POSITIVE WITH IT!

BE IN CHARGE OF YOUR PERSONAL DEVELOPMENT:

1. **STATE YOUR GOALS IN POSITIVE TERMS.** Let those goals be possible and practical; stay away from fantasy. The idea of marrying a wealthy person and spending the rest of your life traveling around the world, while possibly attractive, is not a realistic goal. Your personal goals should stimulate your creativity. **THE IMPORTANT THING IS THAT YOU ARE INSPIRED ABOUT SOMETHING.** Even long term goals have to be worked on day by day. That gives you a reason to get the day started with enthusiasm.

   Stress management consultants all agree that a key element in stress mastery is assessing your personal values and goals. Know where you've been (and learn from your experiences)...where you are...and where you are going. You won't always have it figured out, but the puzzle should be taking shape. If you put pieces here and there without any idea what the puzzle will look like, you might find yourself unhappy with the picture when it is done. The "mid-life crisis" often happens because a person suddenly finds their life half over, and they don't like the picture.

   Only you can maintain and affect the outcome of each goal. Don't make a goal so big you'll give up; achieve it in stages you feel are possible. It keeps you feeling successful rather than discouraged. Don't forget to pat *yourself* on the back with each success.

2. **KNOW WHAT IT WILL TAKE TO MAKE YOU HAPPY.** If you get stuck, you have a choice: DO SOMETHING DIFFERENT! You can only get stuck if you are attached to form, which is your opinion of what's true. Form keeps you inflexible. If you're not attached to inhibiting beliefs, you're available for new experiences (like my raft trip).

YOUR QUEST TO DEVELOP POSITIVE ENERGY WILL BE MORE SUCCESSFUL IF YOU UNDERSTAND YOUR BASIC NEEDS:

* **THE NEED FOR LOVE** - Life's greatest happiness is to be convinced we are loved.

    "THERE IS THE SAME DIFFERENCE IN A PERSON BEFORE AND AFTER HE IS IN LOVE AS THERE IS IN AN UNLIGHTED LAMP AND ONE THAT IS BURNING. THE LAMP IS THERE AND IT WAS A GOOD LAMP, BUT NOW IT IS SHEDDING LIGHT, AND THAT IS ITS REAL FUNCTION."
    - Vincent Van Gogh

* **THE NEED FOR SECURITY** - Too often love is a game with the hope of winning the "big" prize...security. You are the only person you can count on. Develop your own independence because what is true in your life today, may not be true tomorrow.

* **THE NEED FOR RECOGNITION** - Be dynamic; dress to win and turn yourself on!

* **THE NEED FOR NEW EXPERIENCES** - It is this drive that sometimes "makes me wonder why I got myself in this mess." When you stop searching for new experiences in life, you are in the process of dying.

* **THE NEED FOR SELF-ESTEEM** - To feel good about your personal growth and contribution to mankind is as natural a basic need as breathing. Are you just a lamp, or are you giving out light, and being the most you can be?

3. **BE WILLING TO TAKE SENSIBLE RISKS.** Imagine two poles; the left one is where you are, the right one is where you want to be. The space between may be full of worry, fear, and tension (like a big mud puddle you must get dirty to cross). All personal development requires a degree of courage.

> *"NOT RISKING IS THE SUREST WAY OF LOSING. YOU NEVER LEARN WHO YOU ARE, NEVER TEST YOUR POTENTIAL, NEVER STRETCH OR REACH. YOU BECOME COMFORTABLE WITH FEWER AND FEWER EXPERIENCES. YOUR WORLD SHRINKS AND YOU BECOME RIGID. YOU BECOME A VICTIM."* - Dr. David Viscott

There are no failures, only different outcomes. We may feel stupid and ashamed because society is obsessed with success. But, failure is a judgment about an event, and the way we cope with failure is what shapes us - NOT the failure itself. You cannot fail if you accomplish something. It may not be the outcome you originally wanted, but you did not fail if you learned not to do it that way again. Life is one continuous learning process. You look at negative experiences in a new light when you acknowledge they are opportunities for personal growth. . . and you learn . . .and you learn.

4. **KEEP ON OPERATING.** The only way you can fail is to quit! Learn from success AND disappointment; and know that disappointment is not the ONLY response you can have. No one can make you angry, sad, depressed, or discouraged but you. Your reaction is "your" choice! Don't blame anyone else for your choice. You are the one who decides the course of your future.

> *"SUCCESS IS NEVER FINAL, FAILURE IS NEVER FATAL, AND IN DISCOURAGEMENT IS THE WORD 'COURAGE'. IT IS COURAGE THAT COUNTS."*
> - Winston Churchill

Some people might not go to work with a slight headache, but would go on a cruise with the flu. If your intentions are high enough, almost no circumstance will intervene. If your intentions are low enough, any circumstance will intervene.

Sometimes we need a nudge to get going again. This story gives me the perfect word when I need a nudge:

> *A farmer saw a lost horse, and when he got on its back to take it home, he said "giddy-up". The horse chose its own direction, and after a while wandered into the grass. The farmer let the horse eat, then urged the horse to continue down the trail. This happened several times, and each time "giddy-up" was all the horse needed to get back on the path. Eventually, they ended up in the horse's own barn.*

It is alright to wander off the trail occasionally to rest and regenerate. To get anywhere, however, you will need to get back on the trail, and sometimes "giddy-up" is needed to get started again. Staying off the trail to personal development may be comfortable, but it will never be exciting or rewarding.

Until you decide to do something, you'll accomplish nothing. When the alarm goes off in the morning you can think about getting up, say you'll do it and almost get up, but until you put your feet on the floor, you aren't underway! Optimism is fine, but you have to add ACTION. A honeybee may love being a honeybee, but will not make any honey until he makes 3.4 million trips to flowers.

5. **STRETCH SOME ASPECT OF YOUR BEHAVIOR EVERYDAY.** Use someone who is accomplished in your field of interest as a model. It is alright to copy successful techniques.

> *"I WILL PREPARE MYSELF AND PERHAPS MY TIME WILL COME."*   - Abraham Lincoln

6. **USE AFFIRMATIONS TO CHANGE YOUR INTERNAL DIALOGUE TO POSITIVE.** What is true or real is not important. What is important is whether your reality, or life as

you know it, is rewarding to you. The feelings you have, come from what you say to yourself.

7. **LEARN COMMUNICATIONS SKILLS.** Everyone communicates, influences, and manipulates. The question is: How are you going to do it, and for what reason? If you are not getting your point across, you need to understand more about where you are coming from, and also the beliefs of the person to whom you are speaking. Communication means both speaking AND listening.

    A supporting slogan is, "I HAVE AN ABSOLUTE RIGHT TO BE WHO I AM, TO THINK WHAT I THINK, FEEL WHAT I FEEL, AND WANT WHAT I WANT." However, do not confuse "assertiveness" (your right to communicate your feelings) with "aggressiveness" (blaming others and judging their beliefs).

    Knowledge of communication skills can keep you from getting stuck in a conversation that can lead to anger. Anger doesn't deserve to be judged harshly. It is just an emotion, like love, joy, and grief. Emotions are neither good nor bad. It's what you do with them that makes them good or bad!!

    THE TWO MOST COMMON WAYS OF EXPRESSING ANGER IN AN UNHEALTHY WAY ARE:

    - Misdirected anger can cause you to "kick the cat" because you are angry at your spouse. Burying the real problem just creates more problems.

    - Complete suppression is very damaging because once you suppress one emotion, you begin to suppress them all.

    WHEN ANGER IS NOT APPROPRIATELY EXPRESSED, TWO THINGS CAN HAPPEN:

    - Anger may be turned inward and forgotten, leading to ulcers depression, muscle tension, headaches, negative thoughts.

- Anger may "leak out" in indirect ways like accidents, mistakes, poor communication, forgetfulness, procrastination, work blocks, withdrawal, tardiness, and general inefficiency.

8. **PUT YOUR ENERGY INTO CONFIDENCE.** Don't be your own worst enemy. This is a dog-eat-dog world, but it is not the world you are weary of when you have low self-esteem, and feel like a victim. Happiness or misery is a choice you make. *THE MOST DIFFICULT THING PEOPLE HAVE TO LEARN IS THAT YOU CAN'T GO AROUND BLAMING THE WORLD FOR YOUR UNHAPPINESS. IF YOU ARE UNHAPPY - IT IS YOUR CHOICE.* People are always feeling victimized, and are collapsing under the weight of their negative thoughts. It's not stress that is driving you crazy. . .it is your response to stress that makes the difference between "burnout" and "peak performance".

   Accept reality and concentrate on the lessons to be learned. If you give up on yourself, your immune system will too, and you'll get sick! Don't scare yourself, to death with your own negative mental picture. That is wasted energy! Deal with the reality of today and use your energy to improve today. If you interrupt your present negative state, you can alter the outcome of everything that happens in your life, 100% of the time. The situation may stay the same. . .it is your **ATTITUDE** about it that changes.

9. **BE ROMANTIC.** Romance is a passionate commitment to happiness, and keeps you from living automatically. Romance is a right-brain fantasy emotion. To be too romantic is to be too right-brain. To be unromantic is to be too left-brain logical. We need BALANCE for both enjoyment of life and protection of health.

   Being romantic is a lot more than being in love with a person; you can be in love with life. Without loving ourselves or our world, we desperately seek out lust for satisfaction. . .only to find something very important is missing. That frustration makes us angry at ourselves, our world, and the people in it.

10. **GET IN TOUCH WITH THE STATE OF YOUR PHYSICAL HEALTH.** The best mental and emotional suggestions for personal development will fall short of success if you are sick and tired of being sick and tired. So, if you don't want to get that way, the rest of this book is a must to read!

[] [] [] [] [] []

After a personal growth seminar, I wrote this poem about how I felt...

BREAKTHROUGH

I was surrounded by dark walls
    without windows.
The door was closed.
My eyes were open but I could not see.
My mind was closed.
My heart raced with fear and
    insecurity.
My life was closed.
I cried a lot.

The walls are down now.
The light nearly blinds me.
Possibilities are endless.
Frustrations will cease
    with this feeling of peace.
I have forgotten the dark room.
My life is a fresh bloom.
Excitement
Passion
Joy and fun
Look out world...here I come!

Now that you have finished the chapter, you may be thinking that the information sounds good on paper, but wondering if it really works. Believe me, it works...**and keeps working if that is your choice.** Just like you chose to read this chapter, you can choose to make decisions that further your personal growth, and add quality to life.

[] [] [] [] [] []

NOW GO FOR IT!

1. List activities you could enjoy that allow you to participate in life instead of observing.

2. List positive words that can encourage you. Affirm them by repeating them as often as you can.

3. List what isn't working for you. What payoffs are you getting? Remember, a pay-off means something in your subconscious is getting satisfied.

4. List your mindtraps, why you have them, and how they prevent you from dealing with your life in a positive way. Remember, a mindtrap is the way you REACT today to a suppressed fear or negative experience.

5. Determine your current personality group. Determine the personality group of your family members, co-workers, and friends. Assess how this information can improve these relationships.

6. State your goals, how you are stuck, and how you can improve your determination. Revise your goals to realistic levels.

7. List your fears (i.e. I'm not attractive) and then how each fear controls you (i.e. striving for compliments). Decide on some positive affirmations you can repeat often.

8. Acknowledge both positive and negative responses you get from others. Apply what you have learned to improve your own behavior, or increase your self-confidence.

9. Prioritize your problems, and decide on a plan to accept or resolve them.

10. Put some fun, a smile, or a laugh in EVERY DAY!

11. Write your own winning-in-life statement. WHAT DO YOU WANT? Find out what turns your lights on. You know when you've got inner glow, a feeling of self-esteem rooted so deep that nothing can make you doubt yourself.

12. Start each day with a positive attitude.

> *"LET YOUR ENTHUSIASM RADIATE IN YOUR VOICE, YOUR ACTIONS, YOUR FACIAL EXPRESSIONS, YOUR PERSONALITY, THE WORDS YOU USE, AND THE THOUGHTS YOU THINK! NOTHING GREAT WAS EVER ACHIEVED WITHOUT ENTHUSIASM."*
> - Ralph Waldo Emerson

I wrote this one beautiful morning:

**Good morning world!
The sun shines even through the rain.
Drops glisten on my windowpane.
I smile
    and let the day begin.**

"LIFE IS A DARING ADVENTURE, OR IT IS NOTHING."
- Helen Keller

To make your daring adventure healthier. . .read on. . .

CHAPTER 2

NUTRITION

There is a plaque that says, "YOUR HEALTH IS TOO IMPORTANT TO PLACE IN THE HANDS OF YOUR DOCTOR."

Nutrition is not the whole health story, but it is something for which there is no substitute. The several pounds of nutrients you put into your mouth each day are the biggest single determinants of your health.

Americans started the most costly health changes in history when they began living on refined foods, changing from the general use of herbs to synthetic drugs, and decreasing pure water intake for less hydrating and less healthy liquids. Americans cling to the hope that medical science will discover drugs and treatments that will allow them to eat, drink, and be merry while still maintaining good health. THIS HAS BEEN A MYTH FOR YEARS.

Modern health theories have proven to be a disaster to our general health! With infections, epidemics, and injuries being managed well by modern medicine, children and young adults are now suffering from chronic poor health, cancer and other diseases. SOMETHING IS OBVIOUSLY VERY WRONG!!! In an experiment by Frances Pottenger, Jr., M.D. on the effects of diet on lab animals, he concluded that only one generation of processed food produced health changes.

Americans eat far from a balanced diet. Ask any school teacher if they believe diet does not affect mind, and mood. If acknowledged, that could be a powerful beginning to improve our ailing education system. Children with the most refined, junky, and adulterated diets are the ones most likely to goof off, flunk, get sick, or be inconsistent in motivation.

*Most people do not go to the dentist and worry about their **total** health if they have a cavity. They should be aware that A CAVITY IS BODY LANGUAGE THAT THE **BODY IS** NOT HEALTHY . . . NOT JUST THE TOOTH!*

Our health statistics are a national disaster. That is partly due to the fact that healthy diets are a joke. We are the only country in the world where being health conscious makes you a "health nut". One elderly gentleman in a nutrition class defined healthy food by saying, *"If it tastes good, spit it out."* Food taste is a matter of habit; some cultures drink animal blood. You love heavily sugared desserts, fat-marbled meats, and chemical-laden goodies because these are the foods our generation has been taught to enjoy. Habits can be just as easily good, as bad. If you can retrain your taste to enjoy the foods that will build health and not destroy it, you will not have to believe that you won't enjoy the food that provides good nutrition.

Americans are too often motivated by taste appeal, rather than food that we know will improve or maintain our health. We tend not to make *DAILY* dietary choices that protect our *FUTURE HEALTH*. Too many people are indifferent to life. They may not want to die, but when asked about their poor choices say, "You have to die sometime." Without a plan and future goal, people too often live only for immediate pleasures. With our abundance of food we think we are well-fed today. . .or, we will eat better tomorrow. Too often tomorrow is the same fast-paced rat race we had yesterday. It is not the quantities we consume, but our choices of what we eat that are causing nutritional deficiencies in our country today.

We are a well-fed, malnourished society, and health statistics agree. According to the *New Book of World Rankings*, the life expectancy for women in the United States is twelfth place among nations; for men it is seventeenth, for infant mortality we are in twentieth place; on the quality of life index we are in fifteenth place. We are a world leader in many areas, yet our national health statistics are shocking. We have epidemic numbers of cancer, heart disease, high blood pressure, osteoporosis, multiple sclerosis, diabetes, and other diseases that cripple children and adults alike. We eat huge amounts of greasy, salty or sugary *fast food*; highly refined and processed food; and we poison our bodies with caffeine, alcohol, additives and chemicals.

Our poor eating habits have cost us dearly. Health care expenses are rapidly escalating; it is now difficult or impossible for many people to afford needed medical attention. The average person lives with chronic symptoms that reduce the quality of life. Most people only go for medical attention when symptoms become unbearable, or life threatening. To turn current health trends around, we must make dietary changes to practice prevention through healthful living. Never before has there been a greater need for the practice of *"NEWTRITION"* than today!

[] [] [] [] []

THE VILLAINS

You EARN your good health by your willingness to make proper food selections, and eliminate unhealthy habits. If you wish to improve or protect your health you need to stop buying food products that can contribute to illness. For economy you may need to clean up what you've already purchased; you can choose to make better choices when you shop next time. Here are some guidelines for what to avoid:

1. WHITE SUGAR AND EVERYTHING MADE WITH IT:

This does not mean you cannot have your birthday cake, or an occasional social dessert. You make or break your health at home, and it is there you should consume the kind of food that is health building.

Your body needs protein, fat, carbohydrates, vitamins and minerals. Sugar contributes only carbohydrates. Because it goes quickly into the bloodstream raising the blood sugar level and satisfying your appetite, it crowds out your desire to eat other foods that would provide the other nutrition you need.

The whiplash rise and fall in blood sugar on a regular basis overstresses your immune system. Sugar is highly addictive and is the third major component of the American diet, after meat and milk. The top dietary choices are often consumed excessively, and can produce many health problems. It is easier to become addicted to sugar than heroin because of accessibility, cost, and social acceptance.

Do not feel you can improve your health by substituting so called healthier sugars. There is no such thing as a guilt-free goody. All sugar, whether an apple or a candy bar, feeds undesirable intestinal organisms like Candida yeast or parasites. *THE CURE FOR ALL DISEASES* or *THE CURE FOR ALL CANCERS* by Hulda Clark, discusses how parasites can cause any disease in the body.

Sugars other than white refined sugar that may fool you into thinking they are healthier include:

- BROWN SUGAR: This is white refined sugar with a little molasses added. At least use dark brown sugar for a few more nutrients, but don't kid yourself you are improving your health.
- TURBINADO: This is the last stage before white sugar, and is minimally better for you. At best it has fewer chemicals. A cookie jar full of turbinado cookies will feed just as many Candida yeast and parasites as white sugar cookies.
- FRUCTOSE: Mostly derived from corn commercially. One good quality of fructose is that it does not stress the digestive system like white sugar, because it is already a monosaccharide (simple sugar). Unfortunately, it is a chemically refined sugar. Consumed in excess, fructose can increase absorption of triglycerides. Whenever a greater quantity of carbohydrates enter the body than can be immediately used for energy or stored in the liver, the excess is converted to fatty acids called triglycerides. High triglyceride levels have been linked to circulatory diseases.
- SUCANAT: This sugar is naturally dried cane juice made from organically grown sugar cane with all the natural vitamins and minerals. Sucanat is not chemically refined, but some chemicals are needed in the processing. This is better nutritionally, but still keeps your love of sweets in high gear.
- ARTIFICIAL SWEETENERS: The body is not fooled, and gets "quick" sugar one way or another. People using artificial sweeteners often consume too much fruit, fruit juices, refined grains, and sugary treats. Artificial sweeteners are still being studied. Some "safe" choices were proved to be carcinogenic; now the choices are 100 percent safe...until new shocking tests are revealed. We are human guinea pigs for research.

2. TOBACCO

Few people know how tobacco is cured. Our forefathers used natural drying methods, and did not add anything to the tobacco. Many European brands are still using natural drying methods today. Modern American tobacco can be sugar cured; people who smoke are generally unaware of the doubly addictive properties of **both** sugar and tobacco.

Very often in our society, a person who stops smoking increases consumption of candy bars, gum and other sweets in greater quantities than before. They not only have to struggle with the tobacco withdrawal, but they gain weight as well. The sugar in tobacco keeps the blood sugar up so people feel less hungry. Now in a frantic effort for the body to get what it needs, a person may eat continuously because the choices they make are processed foods, not healthy foods.

When you stop smoking, stop eating *ALL REFINED SUGAR, NATURAL SUGAR, AND FRUIT* for two weeks minimum. This allows your body to fight off the allergic hold the sugar had on your system. You'll soon find your sweet cravings less strong. Gradually, you may add tiny amounts of natural sugars and fresh fruit back into your diet, but no refined sugar except for an occasional social situation.

You did not start smoking because it stinks, costs a lot, and can cause serious health problems. So, you will not likely stop for those reasons. Find out the reasons you are blocking or running from life. Deal with it, work through it, and you will likely **want** to make better health choices. Read the Positive Thinking chapter again.

3. TOO MUCH REFINED SALT

Salt is big business! Businesses increase their profit by playing on human addictions to substances like refined salt and refined sugar. Be selective! Select unprocessed foods that you can control refined ingredients. When you prepare from scratch you can add healthier seasalt, and other ingredients.

Organic sodium is a nutrient vital to life. Refined salt (pure sodium chloride) has been heated, and is missing the buffering minerals that make salt a balanced food. This imbalanced product creates health problems; unlike unrefined solar or sun-evaporated seasalt. Solar salt is nature's salt. . .and is good for you in moderation! Healthy salt which is processed only by sun and wind, has a moisture content that contains trace elements essential for health. When the moisture is removed, over seventy valuable trace minerals are lost, and what remains is only sodium chloride. . .an enemy to good health. You get the unhealthy sodium in many ways besides in salt, such as sodium benzoate, sodium nitrate/nitrite, monosodium glutamate, sodium in city water and water softeners.

4. ALL CAFFEINE EXCEPT GREEN TEA

Caffeine is a member of the same addictive alkaloid group of chemicals as morphine, nicotine, cocaine, and purines in meat. People addicted to caffeine may also smoke, crave refined sugar, and eat lots of red meat. Stress and poor dietary choices generally produces a too acid system.

Our caffeine intake is the largest in the world. Besides coffee, caffeine or a similar effect is found in tea, soft drinks, chocolate, and stimulant drugs. The stimulation from caffeine causes the adrenal glands to release hormones that raise the pulse. This signals the liver to release stored sugar; when that sugar reaches the blood it is as much a challenge for the pancreas as consumed sweets. This process robs vitamins, minerals and energy from normal body functions. . .and gives you nothing except added body stress. A few effects from high caffeine use:

- Exhausts pancreas, and can cause hypoglycemia or diabetes.
- Irritates stomach and intestines.
- Imbalances body pH.
- Feeds Candida yeast and parasites if consumed with sugar.
- Stimulates the central nervous system and causes insomnia, nervousness, and fatigue.
- Stimulates the heart and can cause pulse irregularities.
- Increases urination and can cause a loss of nutrients.
- Suspected in breast lumps and birth defects.
* One exception is Green Tea which may be one of the most potent disease preventing substances known. Green Tea has anti-bacterial, anti-viral, anti-fungal, immune stimulating, anti-cancer and circulatory benefits. It is available in both plain, naturally flavored orange or lemon tea, and capsules. Substituting Green Tea for coffee will prevent headache withdrawal symptoms when you attempt to stop coffee.

Commercial concerns have fooled the public into thinking that decaffeinated coffee is a healthful substitute. The chemicals first used to decaffeinate coffee were proven to be carcinogenic. Now, different processes are being used. . .assumed to be 100 percent safe, until perhaps they are later found to be carcinogenic! If you drink decaffeinated coffee on a regular basis, you could be surprised someday that a product you trusted is not safe at all. Do you want to let unproven modern methods determine the quality of your life? There is usually a hidden problem with every modern-day food and drug *breakthrough*. Forgetting *"new and improved"* is a good place to start. The next time you are sitting in a doctor's office, and are sick and tired of being sick and tired, decide if your dietary choices are worth it.

Getting back to basics may be your best defense against poor health. If you insist on drinking an occasional social or morning cup of coffee, purchase unfumigated, unsprayed organic coffee beans from a health food store, and store in the freezer. Grind only enough to consume one cup a day. Ground coffee must be kept in the freezer, because the oils quickly turn rancid. If you drink coffee for an energy lift, you will be better off finding the cause of your fatigue. If you are drinking coffee because you like it, you should look for a healthier substitute like herbal tea, grain coffee substitutes, Green Tea, hot lemon water, blackstrap molasses in hot water, or learn to like plain water. If all other reasoning fails, at least remember **MODERATION**, and for every cup of coffee, drink an extra glass of filtered water.

5. WHITE FLOUR AND EVERYTHING MADE WITH IT

Commercial products are geared more towards profit than nutrition. White flour lasts longer. It is lighter in baking so those products appeal to our modern taste. White flour will not spoil, will not draw bugs and rodents like whole grain flour, and is supposedly "enriched" for your health. It looks like the bugs and rodents are more selective than we are! In refining, about 28 nutrients are removed, and about six synthetic nutrients added. *THIS CAN HARDLY BE CALLED **ENRICHED**.*

White flour is not the *staff of life*. It's empty calories quickly convert to energy, but the body is still waiting for nutrients needed for building and repairing.

Our low-fiber, refined diet acts like glue in the intestines. Modern machinery has taken the outer layer off the grain and removed the germ. Without the germ, flour is a dead food. LIVE FOOD IS FOR LIVE PEOPLE. . .IF MOLD WILL NOT GROW ON IT, NEITHER WILL YOU!

When you read labels look for "whole" wheat as the first word. Commercial labeling is tricky; wheat flour is not whole wheat. Stone ground whole wheat has a higher amount of protein than other processing. Bakery products sold in health food stores will generally have far less chemicals than commercial products, but may still contain refined flour.

6. ALCOHOL - REMEMBER MODERATION

Moderation is as important with alcohol as it is with coffee. An occasional favorite drink may not be a major health issue if you do not feel bad after you drink it, or feel worse the next morning. How you interpret the words "occasional" or "moderation" could be an important factor.

Dealing with emotional issues by strengthening your self confidence and feeling of security, will always be a more healthful approach than escape through alcohol. One drink may not be an overwhelming hazard to your health; but, if you NEED that drink to relax, then you are using alcohol in a harmful way. You should understand whether you are controlling the alcohol, or it is controlling you. The negative effects of daily alcohol consumption are many:

- Changes the body's ability to metabolize zinc, needed in many hormones and enzymes.
- Expands the cells of the intestine so alcohol and food can be absorbed into the bloodstream without complete digestion. *ALCOHOL CONSUMED WITH A MEAL PRODUCES A MUCH GREATER RISK OF ALLERGIC REACTIONS.*
- Supports crutches: not dealing with low self-esteem; not working on poor health that produces symptoms of low blood sugar; not being aware that cravings may be due to allergic withdrawal to grains, sugar, yeast, and certain fruits; not being aware of the dietary demands needed to support Candida Yeast and/or parasite overgrowth.
- Stresses the hardest working organ of your body...your liver. The reasons to "love your liver" are discussed in the Digestion chapter.
- Affects the body the same as sweets. If you are drinking alcohol with sweets, you are giving your body a doubly harmful effect.

7. ALL PROCESSED AND REFINED FOODS

IF IT IS *NEW AND IMPROVED*, FORGET IT! Only natural, unprocessed food can give you a full quota of vitamins and minerals in a state that your body can effectively use.

People can be fooled nutritionally. Soil tests show dramatic differences in mineral content of our agricultural lands. Chemical fertilizers do not replace many of the nutrients taken from the land by continuous cropping.

> *Plants cannot take up nutrients that are not available in the soil, so a crop of peas grown commercially today will not have the same nutritional quality as peas grown a generation ago. Further nutrients are lost in transportation and washing. When the peas are canned, minerals are again lost in the water and some vitamins are affected in various degrees. Heat destroys all enzymes to assist in digestion, so now your body must do all the work. Storage and distribution practices vary, but the canned peas could be several years old when you decide to cook them for dinner. Then you boil the peas and throw the mineral-rich water down the drain, so your unhealthy hydrogenated margarine will stick to them. After the farmer, the packer, the grocer, and you have done your best to eliminate every vestige of nutrition from those peas, you take comfort in having eaten your vegetable for dinner!*

We must stop kidding ourselves that the food we put into our mouths contains all the nutrients we see listed in the food charts. Commercial farming, processing, refining, storage, additives, and cooking all contribute to nutritionally deficient meals. JUST BECAUSE YOU ARE NOT HUNGRY DOES NOT MEAN YOUR CELLS ARE WELL FED! Since you live or die on a cellular level, for good health you must eat food that gives you a fighting chance to be healthy.

Fresh is always best, as long as the fresh is not old and wilted. Dried is second best, because low heat does not destroy enzymes and nutrients like high heat. Mold may be a problem in dried food if you are mold sensitive. Frozen food is next, but should be purchased in a health food store; commercial brands may contain EDTA to preserve freshness that can bind some nutrients, and reduce absorption. Canned food is least nutritious; if eaten, do not through away the liquid. If you have an excess of mineral-rich produce from your organic garden, you may choose to can, but you will preserve more food value if you dry or freeze.

8. EXCESSIVE AMOUNTS OF PROTEIN

Americans eat too much animal protein. The recommended amount of protein varies greatly depending on age, activity, exercise and general health. In spite of our medical research and technological advantages, Americans are a disease-ridden population The average consumption of protein in this country may double or triple the daily needs. . .and that spells ill health in many ways:

- Imbalances the B vitamins. Large amounts of B6 and B3 are needed to metabolize protein.
- Production of ammonia. A dangerous by-product of animal protein metabolism is ammonia, found to be a carcinogenic. There is a high rate of colon and rectal cancer in our meat-eating society.
- Impairment of calcium absorption. The high levels of phosphorus in red meat can cause calcium loss, and may lead to calcium deficiency related diseases such as osteoporosis, osteoarthritis, dental disease, and allergies. In Japan, osteoporosis is low because their diet is low in protein. Calcium balance is determined not only by the amount of calcium you eat, but also by the amount of protein. Excess protein creates acid waste that is neutralized by calcium, depleting it.
- Increased rise in kidney failure. The kidneys excrete protein breakdown products, so high protein intake stresses them.
- Imbalance of acid/alkaline pH. A craving for acid foods can cause addiction to grains, caffeine, carbonated drinks, sugar, alcohol, tobacco, and drugs. An imbalanced pH (discussed in the Digestion chapter) causes people to flock to the drugstore for a barrage of "new and improved" digestive and elimination aids.
- Deficiency of Vitamin A needed to connect amino acids into protein chains.
- Elevates triglyceride levels. When people eat more protein than needed, a large share is stored as fat; a high triglyceride level can be caused by excess protein or carbohydrates.

The body does not store protein as it does fat and carbohydrates, so the food companies have made Americans afraid of getting too little dietary protein. Red meat is a social issue; the more money you make, the more you can afford to eat red meat! Beans are sometimes associated with poverty, and poor quality incomplete protein. Actually, incomplete proteins eaten the *SAME DAY* can *CREATE* complete proteins because we have internal reserves of amino acids to fill in as needed.

Of the 22 amino acids required to build a complete protein, nine cannot be formed by the body, but must be consumed in the diet. No matter what the "eat more meat" advertising tells you, a mixture of animal *AND* vegetable proteins is used most efficiently by the body. Animal protein does not have to be red meat. Hormone and antibiotic-free chicken, turkey, organic eggs, fresh fish and seafood all are easier to digest, and supply needed brain phosphorus not available in vegetable proteins.

Red meat is very hard to digest and puts considerable stress on the liver. Consume red meat in small amounts, not more than twice a week, and always hormone and antibiotic-free. Avoid high-fat, processed, and commercial lunch meats. Do not be fooled with trick advertising:

> *95 percent fat free refers to "weight" of the fat left, and not calories. In 2 percent milk there are five grams of fat and 140 calories per serving. To figure out how many calories in 2 percent milk come from fat, multiply five by nine to convert grams to calories; divide that by total number of calories and you get 45 divided by 140 = 32 percent of the calories come from fat; 2 percent sounds better than 32 percent fat. KEEP TOTAL FAT INTAKE AT OR BELOW 20-25 percent OF CALORIES, AND SATURATED FAT AT 7 percent OF CALORIES OR LESS FOR EACH FOOD ITEM.*

SOME PROTEIN FACTS WORTH KNOWING:

- *Beef eye round is the red meat lowest in fat and cholesterol; always buy hormone and antibiotic-free.*
- *Veal commercially grown should be boycotted, because of the outrageous cruelty to animals, and callous disregard for human health.*

- Lamb is lower in fat because the fat is marbled on the outside and easier to remove. Beef is higher in fat because it is marbled throughout the meat. Lamb has less hormones and antibiotics than other red meats.
- Fish should be rotated to protect against any local pollution problems. Even fresh fish can be shockingly contaminated by bacteria, so rinse in 3% food-grade hydrogen peroxide (as well as meat and fowl), then rinse in water, and wipe dry.
- Animal products are full of antibiotics that imbalance intestinal flora. The influence of hormones given to animals including pork, contributing to our poor health statistics is still being researched. There are some horror stories about the quality used for some commercial products like soup, or cut-up meat products. Purchase organic, or from small market owners dealing with farmers direct, so they know how the animal was raised.
- Eggs should be free range and free of hormones and anti-biotics. An organic egg is a good food because it can produce life; eaten in MODERATION it is a healthy addition to the diet.
- Rabbit is the best animal protein you can eat. It is highest in protein, and lowest in fat and cholesterol of all meats.

9. CHEMICAL FOOD ADDITIVES

IF YOU CAN'T PRONOUNCE IT, DON'T EAT IT! I can pronounce *apple*. Butylated hydrexyanisole, tertiary butylhydroquinone are chemicals used in some salad dressings, that don't sound like words said around the old country wood stove.

It's quite a surprise when you read lists of ingredients on the packages of highly processed foods in your grocery store. They look like shopping lists for chemists! I live simply . . . back to basics. I have absolute standards for the food I purchase for my home. When I go to a restaurant, I order sensibly, or even indulge occasionally; the rule is, YOU MAKE OR BREAK YOUR HEALTH AT HOME. I'm never tempted to purchase products that contain preservatives, artificial coloring or flavoring, nitrates or nitrites, monosodium glutamate, refined sugar or flour, EDTA, or other additives. We are told these chemicals are perfectly safe, but current health statistics suggest something is very wrong. Consumers need to continue demanding healthier food! The products you choose to purchase has tremendous power!!!

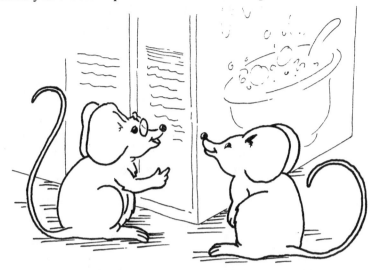

We're not touchin' any of this stuff
until we find something NUTRITIOUS!

One organization that deserves credit for studying the effects of chemicals in our diet is the Feingold Association. Their research has shown a connection between hyperactivity in children and consumption of food additives and sugar. Many hyperactive children turn into irritable, nervous adults. The Feingold information can help all ages. A call to your school board should get you in touch with your local organization.

Eat simple unprocessed, non-chemical whole foods in their natural, uncomplicated form. Chemicals have only been in existence since World War II. Considering the appalling health of the general population it is hard to believe our bodies can adjust so quickly to so many invasive changes. Truth is. . .it hasn't. But, disease is BIG BUSINESS!

10. SATURATED FAT AND HYDROGENATED OILS

FATS FALL INTO THREE CATEGORIES:

- highest in saturated fats are red meat, coconut and palm oils, and lard; these harden at room temperature

- highest in monounsaturated fats are flaxseed, olive, almond, avocado, canola and peanut oils; these are liquid at room temperature
- highest in polyunsaturated fat are safflower, sunflower, soy and corn oils; also liquid at room temperature

Knowing what to pick is based on the oil's ability to change to trans-fatty acid formation. Trans-fatty acids are unnatural to the body and bad for your health. Monounsaturated fats are not subject to as much trans-fatty acid formation, so oils high in monounsaturated fats are the current health trend. Because of this trend, mono-rich safflower, corn and sunflower oils are all being developed. Both consumer and manufacturer may win since monounsaturated oils are more stable.

Polyunsaturated oils first became popular because of their ability to lower serum cholesterol. They are nutritious and beneficial when fresh, but are especially subject to attack by oxygen. Outside your body this means oil becomes rancid; inside the body it undergoes a similar change forming free radicals that may lead to disease. Another problem is polyunsaturated fats also reduce HDL levels, the good cholesterol. Monounsaturated oils lower LDL cholesterol too, but have a neutral effect on HDL cholesterol.

When Americans started to understand the relationship between fats and health, the wonderful commercial industries had to do something fast. They could not protect their investment if chosen oils turned rancid. They had to "invent" an oil that would act like a saturated fat, but the label could read *no saturated fat*. In their infinite wisdom they came up with hydrogenated oils. Don't be fooled by modern science. Remember, IF IT'S NEW AND IMPROVED, THE MANUFACTURERS MAY SMILE ALL THE WAY TO THE BANK, BUT IT MAY NOT GOOD FOR YOUR HEALTH!

> ***Unsaturated*** *fats can be converted into **saturated** fats by a process called **hydrogenation** so they won't become rancid during frying or while being stored. This process acts like a chemical hair-straightener, turning natural, curved unsaturated fatty acids into straight man-made trans-fatty acids. Hydrogenated oils in margarine, vegetable shortening, and most processed foods and snacks are so destructively*

altered they are worse for your health than saturated animal fats. Until the government is willing to unchain themselves from the politics of the food industry, facts will continue to be blocked from the consumer.

Hydrogenation produces high levels of trans-fatty acids, which intensify essential fatty acid deficiencies, and produces "weird prostaglandins." Your health depends on the presence of short-lived cellular hormones (some live only a few seconds) called prostaglandins, to act as chemical catalysts in every activity that goes on in your body every second of your life. Your body does not make prostaglandins. They are made by the breakdown process of the essential fatty acids in foods like whole grains, nuts and seeds, and cold-pressed oils. Refining removes the "life" part of the oil, and all that is left is the fat.

Always buy cold-pressed oils because they have not been refined, and still contain the essential fatty acids needed by your body. IF AN OIL WILL NOT TURN RANCID, IT WILL NOT DO YOU ANY GOOD! Again, new and improved is generally not healthier!

All vegetable oils are cholesterol-free. Labeling laws have improved, but often the details are overlooked with packaging headlines like "Made with 100 percent vegetable oil" or *no cholesterol.* These products may contain tropical or hydrogenated oils. You need to read ALL the package information.

11. MILK AND DAIRY PRODUCTS

"Modern" milk is not the same milk your grandparents consumed, and has no right being called a perfect food by today's standards. Milk is hard to digest; mucus forming; and may contain hormones, antibiotics, chemicals, drugs, pesticides, and radioactive strontium from the atmosphere. It has been linked to many physical symptoms such as:

- colic in babies, and intestinal problems in adults
- diarrhea, and iron deficiency
- sinus, ear, respiratory symptoms in children and adults
- headaches

- chronic joint pains
- cold extremities

THERE ARE SOME FACTS ABOUT MILK YOU SHOULD KNOW:

- We are the only mammals on the earth drinking another mammals milk by choice, and regularly drinking it as adults. Goat's milk is better than cow's milk because it is closer to the composition of human milk. It should be the first choice for babies if mother's milk is not available.
- Our ability to digest milk sugar (lactose) decreases after about age four. Chronic intestinal problems are often linked to the inability to digest milk sugar. Pasteurization inactivates natural digestive enzymes in milk making it hard to digest. The new ultra-pasteurization destroys even more nutrients. . .the shelf life is extended, but at what cost to our health?
- It is surprising how apparent it is that cow's milk can produce disease, and yet it is politically protected by the government, buying and stockpiling excess to prevent price fluctuations.
- Dr. Kurt Oster, a cardiologist, believes homogenized milk releases an enzyme called Xanthine Oxidase, that is absorbed through the intestinal wall, circulates in the blood, and is deposited in the blood vessel wall. Here this lethal enzyme may create the beginning of plaque formation and arteriosclerosis. *THE MILK BOOK* by William Campbell Douglass discusses this process, and other ways science has destroyed this natural food. Heart attacks are fewer in countries where milk is not homogenized. Milk is first pasteurized, then homogenized (fat broken up under pressure); most milk products are made from homogenized milk. Heat kills Xanthine Oxidase, but after pasteurization 40 percent of Xanthine Oxidase still remains. Further cooking of milk in recipes would be better in this instance.
- Cow's milk has 1200 milligrams of calcium per quart, human milk has 300 milligrams, yet an infant on human milk absorbs more calcium. . .WHY? Calcium to phosphorus ratio should be 2-1 or more. Too much phosphorus can reduce calcium absorption. Cow's milk ratio is 1.2-1, human milk ratio is better than 2-1.
- Then there is the all-American ice cream. . .not what Grandma used to make. Ice cream manufacturers are not required by law to

list the additives, and the same additives may also be used in some household and industrial products, like paint remover, leather cleaner, lice killer, antifreeze and coal tar. DELICIOUS MAY NOT BE NUTRITIOUS!

[] [] [] [] [] []

THE HEROES

WE ARE A SICK-ORIENTED SOCIETY THAT THINKS WE CAN EAT, DRINK, AND BE MERRY BECAUSE THE MEDICAL PROFESSION WILL SAVE US. THE TRAINING MOST AMERICANS GET ON HEALTH AWARENESS IS LIKE PUTTING OUT A HOUSE FIRE WITH A SQUIRT GUN. WE TREAT OURSELVES FOR PHYSICAL, EMOTIONAL, AND MENTAL SYMPTOMS, AND ESCAPE INTO ADDICTIVE HABITS BECAUSE WE CANNOT HANDLE OUR STRESSFUL WORLD.

Health metamorphosis occurs when the human body gets what it needs to work at optimum performance. . .the body heals itself. Here are some basic healthy food tips. . .THINK HEALTH, NOT DISEASE!

"Let nature be your teacher."
- Wordsworth

1. NATURAL SUGARS

The sweeteners with some nutritional value are sorghum, honey, maple syrup, and blackstrap molasses. Even these sugars should be eaten in small amounts. I talked to one lady who proudly proclaimed that she did not let her son use any refined sugar, and she wondered if a half cup of honey on his cereal was too much! People who are used to consuming large amounts of refined sugar think they are eating better when they consume just as much natural sugar. Having an assortment of cookies, cakes, pies, and sweet breads always on hand keeps you addicted to sweet foods, whether they were made with refined or natural sugar. Learn to reduce your need for sweet taste.

A FEW FACTS ABOUT NATURAL SUGARS YOU SHOULD KNOW:

HONEY should be raw, unrefined, unfiltered, and unheated. Honey is high in fructose, which does not need insulin to break it down. Since fructose is already a simple sugar, it is less of a digestive strain than refined sugar. Tupelo honey from Florida and Blackbutton Sage honey are both high in fructose compared to other honeys. The cheapest honey is bought on tap. Mild honey is light in color and taste; darker honeys are stronger flavored, and richer in minerals.

There are many excellent books on cooking, eating, and canning with honey. I want to emphasize that occasional "treat" recipes add fun to life. I do not use sweet dinner recipes, but the following is a favorite "party" snack that can be enjoyed occasionally, because you eat right most of the time:

Purchase 12-14 dejointed chicken wings; trim skin as much as possible, pat dry and place in casserole. Mix 1/2 cup honey with 3 tablespoons cornstarch or arrowroot, 1/2 teaspoon ginger, 1/2 cup water, 1/3 cup fresh squeezed lemon juice, 1/4 cup soy sauce. Cook until thickened, pour over wings and bake at 350 degrees for 45 minutes, turning several times. Place on stove top and cook 15 minutes stirring almost constantly to boil down liquid and glaze - ENJOY!

MAPLE SYRUP is between 60 to 65 percent sucrose (white sugar is 99 percent sucrose, honey rarely over 3 percent). The rest is water and minerals. Pure maple syrup can contain dangerous amounts of lead, leached from metal buckets with lead solder. Holes drilled in trees are often kept open with paraformaldehyde pellets. This practice is unlawful in Canada so I always buy Canadian maple syrup; some New England producers avoid it voluntarily, and will provide affidavits to this effect. Health food stores offer safe maple syrup, which is less expensive if bought on tap.

BLACKSTRAP MOLASSES is a by-product of the cane sugar industry. Blackstrap is the first stage in cane sugar refining, and should be chosen over other types of molasses. It is an excellent source of the B vitamins, iron, calcium, potassium, and trace minerals. It is 65 to 70 percent sucrose. One tablespoon of blackstrap molasses in a cup of hot water makes a great mineral drink, and is a natural laxative. I have a favorite bran muffin recipe that uses blackstrap molasses:

Soak 1 cup bran in 1 cup soy or rice milk (do not pack) for 5 minutes. Add 1 egg, 1/4 cup cold-pressed oil, 2 full tablespoons blackstrap molasses, and beat well. Mix 1 1/2 cups whole wheat flour, 3 teaspoons baking powder, 1/2 level teaspoon sea salt together; stir into the bran mixture. Bake at 400 degrees for 25-30 minutes in 12 PAM sprayed muffin cups.

SORGHUM is an edible tropical grass seed that produces a sweet juice. It is 65 to 70 percent sucrose.

STEVIA is a natural non-caloric sweetener 200 times sweeter than sugar, and safe even for Candida yeast or parasite overgrowth. Your health food store may need to order it for you.

2. SUN-EVAPORATED OR SOLAR SEA SALT

The Grain and Salt Society (address in reference section) sells an excellent informative book, and totally natural sea salt (Celtic Salt) from the ocean. This completely unrefined salt possesses the power to restore wholeness and balance to our body fluids. DO NOT TAKE THIS RECOMMENDATION CASUALLY. HEALTH MEANS INTERNAL BALANCE!!!

DeSouza's Solar Sea Salt is available in coarse, fine and extra fine salt from health food stores, or DeSouza's Food Corporation, P.O. Box 395, Beaumont, CA 92223. It is less refined than other commercial sea salts, but a second choice over the naturally harvested, chemical-free, and perfectly balanced Celtic Sea Salt. **Some sea salt is too refined; it must say solar or sun-evaporated, not just sea salt.**

3. WHOLE GRAINS

Whole grains are rich in fiber and nutrients. They are complex carbohydrates, so they break down slowly in the digestive process, and do not saturate the system with simple sugar like refined sugars, fruits, dairy products, and refined grains.

Grains need to be either cooked or sprouted for best nutritional absorption. Sprouted grains and unleavened bread are good for yeast sensitive people. Grind grains fresh before using, or buy in small amounts and store in the refrigerator. Whole grains, unlike processed and refined grains, will turn rancid with age. Your overworked liver will have to deal with the problem. If the good oils are removed to protect against rancidity, the food does not contain the "good stuff" you need for health. REFINED FOOD IS DEAD FOOD!

Develop your taste for *ALL* the whole grains, not just wheat. Grains high in gluten (which cause some people to experience stomach and intestinal complaints) are wheat, oats, rye, barley, spelt, and a non-grain buckwheat which has a gluten-like protein. Spelt is the most tolerated grain, even for some gluten sensitive people. Health food stores have a full range of bakery items made with spelt; they also carry baked goods with less chemicals and sometimes organically grown ingredients.

There are other ways to manage meals without the usual bread:

Celery, green or red bell peppers, tomatoes, organic potato skins, romaine lettuce leaves, fresh or wilted cabbage or chinese cabbage leaves can all hold sandwich ingredients.

Spaghetti squash is a great substitute for wheat spaghetti: Boil spaghetti squash in water to cover, for about 40 minutes, depending on size. Split in half and flip out spaghetti-like strands with a fork. Serve with your favorite sauce.

Non-gluten grains are rice, corn, and millet. Rice cakes and corn tortillas are good bread substitutes for the gluten intolerant. Millet is the forgotten grain although it has been used for 1500 years. It is unfortunate its birdseed appearance has prevented its popularity, because it is one of the most nutritious foods known to man, and the most nutritious grain. Millet and cooked carrots are good for diarrhea. A macrobiotic cooking class taught me how to make millet delicious:

Cook one cup millet in three cups slightly salted water for 20 minutes; drain. Place one inch of water in a steamer. Cover millet with a towel before placing lid on. As it steams, the towel absorbs the moisture so it does not drip into the millet. The millet puffs up like popcorn into a delicious grain.

Any grain can be an allergic food. If you have any unexplained chronic symptom, and you crave any grain product, you should suspect an allergy to the grain you eat most often. To test a grain (or any food):

***COMPLETELY** avoid all grains (or other food being tested) for four days. During this period it is not uncommon to have withdrawal symptoms of any flu-like nature, or an aggravated version of an existing symptom. Symptoms usually clear by the end of the third day. On the fifth day of withdrawal, pick a time that allows at least two free hours, and **at least one hour when you can sit down**. Record how you feel, and record your pulse taken at your wrist for one full minute; then eat a small portion of the food to be tested. Record symptoms and pulse at 20, 40, and 60 minutes after eating. A pulse increase or decrease of eight points, or symptoms, indicates a probable sensitivity. If there are no symptoms eat a second portion of the same food and evaluate symptoms in 30 and 60 minutes. You may be surprised at how a "healthy food" is the cause of your discomfort.*

Two of my favorite grain recipes are:

- *French toast made with 4 slices of any whole grain bread: whip 2 organic eggs, add 1/8 cup rice or soy milk, 1 teaspoon cinnamon, 1/4 teaspoon seasalt (adjust ingredients according to taste); brown, and top with Better Butter (recipe on page 63) and pure maple syrup.*

- *Whole wheat pancakes made with whole wheat or spelt flour: separate two organic eggs and whip whites into stiff peaks. Place yolks in a larger bowl and add 1 cup of flour, 1 cup rice or soy milk, 1 tablespoon cold pressed Canola oil (or any other cold pressed oil except olive), 2 teaspoons pure maple syrup to help brown,*

1/2 teaspoon seasalt, 1 1/2 teaspoons aluminum-free baking powder. Blend all ingredients, and fold in egg whites. May add 1 cup fresh blueberries if desired. Bake on griddle sprayed with PAM; top with pure maple syrup, optional Better Butter. . .ENJOY!

4. VEGETABLES

I can almost guarantee you that if you eat lots of raw vegetables and drink eight glasses of filtered water for a month (no dairy or red meat, refined sugar or refined grains), you'll notice a distinct change in the way you feel. Vegetables are low in carbohydrates, high in vitamins, minerals, enzymes, aid in digestion, assist in keeping the system from becoming too acid, and are the "regenerators" of the body. If your vegetables are not organic, you should add a liquid mineral supplement available from health food stores.

However, when introducing new foods to your family, cook QUIETLY! You don't have to announce that the family spaghetti sauce contains wheat germ. Shock treatment of making a friend's favorite blueberry pie with whole wheat crust and honey is not the place to start teaching healthier eating. New vegetables may meet shocking resistance. At one family meal, I served soup with seaweed in it. My son asked, "What's that green stuff floating around in my soup?" When I explained that it was seaweed, my husband said, "You had to ask?" Changing the family diet is like breaking ground. . .one shovelful at a time.

Most vegetables should be eaten raw except rhubarb, beans, peas, potatoes, and corn (a grain). Some vegetables like spinach, asparagus, cauliflower, cabbage and broccoli are high in phytates, which if eaten raw all the time, can decrease the availability of the nutrients in those foods. They are best steamed, or eaten raw in moderation.

Chopping exposes cut surface to air causing oxidation, which destroys nutrients like Vitamin A, C, B6, thiamine and biotin. Do not prepare cut vegetables ahead of time, purchase food at grocery salad bars, or purchase packaged precut vegetables. A lot of nutrients are concentrated in the outer layer, so scrub instead of peel if organic. If the nonorganic food looks shiny (like apples and cucumbers), they are covered with a hydrocarbon wax, and should be peeled.

Give your vegetables proper care after you buy them. Bring them straight home, wash them VERY WELL in Shaklee Basic-H organic cleanser, Amway L.O.C., or a fruit and vegetable wash from a health food store; store them in sealed glass jars or zip lock bags in the refrigerator. One shelf in my refrigerator contains nothing but glass containers with all my vegetable selections. Vegetables stay fresh longer in glass than in the vegetable bin, and do not lose their nutrients as quickly. All food begins to lose nutrients as soon as the food is harvested; fresh fruits and vegetables are especially perishable, so take care to minimize this deterioration.

Don't be afraid to try new vegetables. People tend to buy the same vegetables week after week. This book is not intended to be a cookbook of recipes. There are many good health cookbooks available in health food stores, and you should purchase several. These two suggestions are DELICIOUS and may introduce you to several new vegetables:

Once the woody peel is cut off jicama, you have a delicious vegetable, cooked or raw as finger food. Shoestring jicama looks and tastes like potatoes. Peel and thinly slice one jicama into strips. In 1 tablespoon sesame oil sauté jicama, two cloves crushed garlic, 3 tablespoons chopped red bell pepper, 1/8 teaspoon paprika, and 1/8 teaspoon seasalt for 10 minutes (stir frequently). Lightly top with fresh ground black pepper. This is a delicious and unique substitute for potatoes.

Kohlrabi is another unusual vegetable, delicious cooked in salted water for 15 minutes or more, or eaten raw. It is an odd-looking light green vegetable with leaves growing out of a bulblike stem. The name means cabbage-turnip in German. It is great raw finger food, cut into slivers and put in a salad, or as part of a platter of vegetables and a zingy dip.

Steaming (drink mineral-rich liquid left in pan), stir frying, or waterless cooking are best ways to cook vegetables because nutrients are not lost in discarded water. Soup is a good mineral rich food. Cooking in a pressure cooker has been forgotten in recent years. This is a shame because protein, starches and vegetables cook up quickly and taste naturally sweet. Pressure cooking allows you to use less frequently consumed root vegetables. A delicious dinner (including the liquid) is:

> *One hormone and antibiotic-free skinned chicken. Add a combination of carrots, onions, cabbage, potatoes, parsnips, or turnips as desired. Salt with seasalt. Water and cooking time is based on the book that comes with the cooker.*

Microwave ovens are advertised to retain nutrients, but cooking may change the molecular structure adversely. I no longer choose to experiment with my life using modern technology, or "new and improved" products. I'm most comfortable going back to basics since *all* the data will take many years to compile, and may still be missing important health statistics. I heat in my microwave, but never cook longer than two minutes. NEVER heat water in the microwave in a ceramic cup as it can leach out lead. NEVER STAY IN FRONT AND LOOK AT A MICROWAVE OVEN WHEN IT IS RUNNING.

Learn to be a bean lover! Legumes are high in fiber, protein, many necessary nutrients, low in fat and provide recipes that keep you from eating so much red meat. Many people avoid them because of their gas-forming properties (indigestible sugars that the body cannot break down). If you prepare your beans correctly, you can enjoy them without distress:

> *Soak overnight or 4-6 hours and discard the water. This soaking may be enough to eliminate problems; if not try this next step. Cover with water and bring to a boil; boil one minute and discard that water. The beans can then be boiled until they are well done, in the amount of water that is not completely absorbed. Always discard the cooking water before using the beans in your favorite recipes. Cooked beans freeze well; make enough for multiple quick meals.*

> *If you cook black-eyed peas, you can freeze them in serving sizes, thaw as desired and toss with cold-pressed mayonnaise and chopped white onions. If you cannot tolerate onions, add any desired vegetable, like tomatoes or cucumber to cooked beans and mayonnaise.*

5. FRUIT

The best way to eat fruit is in small amounts, in season, and raw. Fruit is high in simple carbohydrates. Your health will not improve as quickly as you wish if you switch from junk food sweets to a "fruitaholic or juiceaholic" diet. Candida yeast and parasites thrive on the breakdown process of sugar either from unhealthy candy bars or healthy apples. Fresh fruit is best eaten no more than once or twice daily. It takes too much fruit to make a glass of juice. . .your Candida yeast and parasites can have a birthday party from all the simple sugar.

Orange juice does not contain the valuable bioflavonoids found in the white membrane; you don't get the food value of the entire orange. Next time you feel like having a glass of orange juice, eat an orange and drink a glass of water! Tremendous quantities of fiber are thrown away when apple juice is processed. I buy grapes instead of grape juice, and never the seedless variety; there is valuable nutrition in those fibrous seeds!

The best fruits are not excessively sweet. Tart apples, cherries, strawberries, papaya, grapefruit, lemon, and pineapple are all good selections. Seasonal fruit that is naturally ripened and contains a large stone or pit is easily digested and absorbed by the body. Dates, mangoes, papayas, apricots, peaches, avocados, cherries, plums, prunes, and grapes with seeds are all excellent. Naturally ripened fruit is not always easy to find; if you can buy fruit directly from the grower, in season, you have a better chance of getting full nutritional value.

6. FATS AND OILS

Fats, proteins and carbohydrates are the primary sources of energy for the body, supplying fuel for body heat and physical activity. "Calorie" is a term that signifies the amount of energy that is released as heat when food is metabolized. Fats are high caloric foods and yield about nine calories per gram; protein and carbohydrates yield four calories per gram.

A low-fat diet is important to your health in many ways. When you consume fat, it should do you some good. The best oils are cold-pressed. The essential fatty acids that break down to produce chemicals called prostaglandins are preserved by the cold-pressing process. Refrigerate all open bottles because "alive" oils can turn rancid.

The two most important fatty acids in human nutrition are linoleic acid from Omega 6 oils and linolenic acid from Omega 3 oils which the body cannot make. The best sources for both are Black Currant Seed oil,

Hemp oil, and Flaxseed oil. Flaxseed oil needs sulfurated protein to completely break it down in the system, so for improved absorption it should be taken with soy milk, rice milk, or whole wheat bread. Fish oil is just Omega 3, and Evening Primrose is just Omega 6. Research has shown the best therapeutic value is in receiving both.

DO NOT ELIMINATE ESSENTIAL FATTY ACIDS IN YOUR EFFORT TO REDUCE FATS! ESSENTIAL FATTY ACIDS ARE NEEDED FOR HEALTHY GLANDULAR FUNCTION. . ..A BIG MISTAKE TO ELIMINATE THEM!

Fatty acids are destroyed easily by heat, light, and oxygen, so a diet high in processed foods will be deficient in essential fatty acids. It is best to consume good fats and oils in the form of whole, unprocessed foods such as raw nuts and seeds, whole grains, and cold-pressed oils; and/or take an essential fatty acid supplement.

Sesame oil is best for frying because it does not break down into carcinogenic free radicals as rapidly as other oils when it is heated. Olive oil is good for the liver; use it in salad dressings, with fish or seafood, and in stir frying as often as possible. Olive oil is about 75% monounsaturated fats. Virgin has the most olive taste; then comes extra fine virgin; then refined, from olives too acidic, or having an "off" flavor. Pure olive oil is a mixture of refined and virgin oils. "Light" is pure olive oil with less virgin oil for only a hint of olive taste, so it is most popular for general cooking. All olive oil is best for the liver; the least refined is always best. Virgin olive oil will harden in the refrigerator, so I always transfer it into a wide mouth jar so I can take out what I want easily.

Use organic butter instead of margarine. I do not recommend hydrogenated margarine because it is high in free radicals that can be carcinogenic, and margarine can block the body's production of prostaglandins. Foods in their natural form are always healthier than processed foods. Butter is rich in a form of Vitamin A that is 300% more than the Vitamin A in fish liver oil. Natural D in butter is equal to 10 quarts of milk and 100 times as effective as a synthetic form. Vitamin F in butter acts like a partner with Vitamin D. Vitamin E in butter is a whole, natural complex. *BUTTER IN MODERATION IS A GOOD FOOD, BUT "BETTER BUTTER" IS LOWER IN SATURATED FAT*

AND HIGHER IN ESSENTIAL FATTY ACIDS. The following recipe stays soft in the refrigerator, and tastes delicious:

> *1 pound organic butter - very soft*
> *1 cup water*
> *1 cup cold-pressed canola oil*
> *Blend in a heavy-duty mixer (not a light blender), food processor, or use a hand mixer. Place in a closed container and refrigerate. You can make one half recipe and freeze two sticks of butter for later, if you use butter infrequently.*

If you have a milk allergy, sinus or respiratory mucus problems, you should be able to use butter because the allergic properties are not in the fat, nor is butterfat mucus forming.

Do not save and reheat any type of oil. I do not recommend deep fat frying for any food, but if you love French fries, try these three recipes:

> *- For EACH unpeeled potato: slice like French fries, coat with 2 teaspoons of sesame tahini, and 1/4 teaspoon seasalt. Place on oiled baking sheet and bake 35-40 minutes at 450 degrees, turning several times.*
>
> *- Cut 2 potatoes into 8 lengthwise wedges; soak in cold water 30 minutes; pat dry. Toss with 1 tablespoon olive oil, 2 teaspoons oregano leaves, 1/4 teaspoon seasalt; lay out single layer on baking pan. Bake 400 degree oven 35-40 minutes until potatoes are tender and brown; turn once. Sprinkle with fresh ground black pepper, and 2 tablespoons malt vinegar.*
>
> *- 2 small sweet potatoes, peeled*
> *1 Tablespoon olive oil*
> *1/8 teaspoon cayenne*
> *1/4 teaspoon seasalt*
> *Heat oven to 450 degrees. Cut potatoes into 3 inch long matchstick shapes. Place in a bowl and pour the olive oil over potatoes; sprinkle with cayenne and seasalt. Using your hands, toss the potato sticks until completely coated with oil. Spread out in a single layer on a baking*

> sheet. Bake about 25 minutes, turning every 10 minutes or so. The sweet potatoes are done when they are tender and almost caramelized; they won't really crisp up like french fries but will have a chewy sweetness.

7. PROTEIN

It is important that you put protein in perspective, both in quantity and quality in your diet. Your protein does not have to be hard-to-digest red meat. A serving of red meat several times a week, or in a soup base is all you should consider, and indeed more than you need. Eat more fish, hormone and antibiotic-free fowl, rabbit, and moderate numbers of organic eggs; or add Braggs Liquid Aminos as a delicious source of life-renewing protein (health food stores, or 1-800-446-1990). Most of us need to greatly reduce our consumption of meats, but not everyone should be a vegetarian.

> *Dr. William Donald Kelly devised a test to determine an individual's energy needs and the kinds of protein best suited for their specific body chemistry: Take a 50 milligram niacin tablet on an empty stomach first thing in the morning. If a flush of uncomfortable degree (or maybe even hives) develops, that person can handle the digestion of sensible amounts of animal protein. If the tablet produces just a mild warm feeling, the person can eat occasional meat. If no reaction occurs, the diet would be better vegetarian. This test may change as your health changes.*

A person does not have to eat red meat, but some vegetarians get very tired if they do not consume a little chicken, eggs, fish, or seafood. THE DECIDING FACTOR IS HOW DO YOU FEEL ON YOUR CURRENT DIET? If you are eating animal products, or you are a strict vegetarian, this test might show you that you are consuming a diet that does not meet your body's needs.

HERE ARE SOME FACTS ON PROTEIN CHOICES:

- **Fish** contains an Omega 3 fatty acid that is not found in significant amounts in any other food. It keeps the protein in your blood from becoming sticky and forming clots. People living in coastal countries and Eskimos statistically have fewer heart attacks. You should eat fish at least three times a week. If you do not enjoy fish, substitute a supplement that contains Omega 3 fatty acid. You should also know that the reason you don't think you like fish is that you may not be fixing it correctly. Overdone, tough and oily tasting fish, is not delicious. Try some of my favorite ideas:

a. *Freshly broiled salmon cooked until it flakes but still has moisture, and the deep pink color is gone. Chinook salmon is higher in fat than silver salmon. Sauté or bake salmon in a little Better Butter and chopped spring onions. Bake at 350 degrees for 10-15 minutes only. Canned salmon makes great salmon salad, salmon cakes, or salmon loaf.*
b. *Haddock is one of the tastiest of the firm white fish; be careful NOT to overcook. Many people do not like fish because it is dry and overcooked. Fix haddock the same as you would salmon.*
c. *Clam chowder can be made "milk" free with a non-dairy milk, or with a tomato base. Use clam sauce on whole wheat spaghetti or spaghetti squash for a change. Clam sauce is easy to make:*

> Sauté 2 large chopped garlic cloves and 2 tablespoons chopped onion in 1/8 cup olive oil until soft. Add 1/4 cup whole wheat flour, 2 teaspoons basil, 1 bottle clam juice, 2 rounded tablespoons fresh parsley, and cook until thickened. Add 2 cans minced clams with juice (read labels - find one without sugar), and 1/4 teaspoon seasalt; heat only - boiling toughens clams. Top with fresh, chopped spring onions and soy parmesan cheese.

d. *Bouillabaisse, or fisherman's soup, is a sure hit at dinner; the recipe is in fish cookbooks. Bottled clam juice and fish fillets turn vegetable soup into bouillabaisse.*

e. *Sauté any fish fillet and serve on a whole wheat hamburger roll; use your imagination for the garnishings for your own **fabulous fish burger**.*

f. If you wish to sauté razor clams, pound the necks with a mallet and cook in a little Better Butter for 30 seconds on a side; they will toughen if overcooked.
g. One of my favorite fish recipes:

> Arrange six lightly salted large sole fillets in a single layer on a baking dish sprayed with **PAM**. Top with a mixture of 1/2 cup cold-pressed oil mayonnaise and 2 teaspoons natural mustard. Bake at 350 degrees for 10-15 minutes depending on thickness of sole.

h. *Fried seafood is not recommended. It is high in fat, and restaurant fried food could be in rancid oil. The only fried food I eat is an occasional treat of tiny fried oysters, coated with a little sea salt and whole wheat flour, browned over medium heat in cold-pressed sesame oil.*
i. If you do not like plain sardines, add to tomato soup.
j. Fish fillets can be fixed in a variety of ways to satisfy even the skeptical fish eater. Cut fish fillets into 1 inch chunks and check for bones. Place in a casserole sprayed with PAM, and let your imagination CREATE a sauce:

- Wine, Worcestershire sauce and lime juice
- Mayonnaise and mustard
- Your favorite **BBQ** sauce
- Curry, Better Butter, and almonds
- Lemon, Better Butter and herbs like basil, sage, thyme, marjoram, parsley, chives
- Better Butter, fresh parsley, lemon and fresh grated ginger root
- Leftover vegetarian spaghetti sauce
- Pesto sauce (from health food stores)
- Your favorite salad dressing
- Soy sauce, wine vinegar and lemon juice
- Fresh grated ginger and soy sauce
- Sauté olive oil, onion, garlic, celery, tomato until tender, then add to fish
- Garlic, lemon juice, Dijon mustard, Better Butter; top with fresh ground pepper

BE CREATIVE! *Bake in a preheated 350 degree oven for 10-15 minutes depending on the thickness of the chunks. Do not overcook! Be willing to try every kind of fish and seafood, and be surprised by new taste treats!*

- **Chicken** should be skinned, hormone and antibiotic-free. White meat is lower in fat than dark meat. Think plain! There are many chicken recipes that do not use lots of fat, dairy, or sugar in sauces. Any combination under "j." for fish can also be used for chicken. Here is a recipe for a good non-creamy sauce:

    Skin 4 chicken breasts and low-heat sauté in 1 tablespoon cold-pressed sesame oil with 1 sliced onion. Add 1 can natural chicken broth available at a health food store; season with 1/2 teaspoon each marjoram, basil, thyme, and tarragon, 1-2 teaspoons curry (to taste), and 1 tablespoon parsley. Cook about 45 minutes, or until chicken is done. Thicken with cornstarch or arrowroot; serve sauce over brown rice.

    This is great for special occasions: Skin one chicken (or use desired parts), sauté in 1/4 cup cold-pressed sesame oil, 1 small chopped onion, 2 large garlic cloves, 1/2 teaspoon seasalt, 1 ROUNDED tablespoon oregano leaves, on **medium-low** *heat 45 minutes - 1 hour; turn occasionally. Remove chicken; stir into sauce 1 fresh tomato cut in wedges per person, just to coat with juices but not to cook. Serve with tomatoes around chicken on a platter. . . beautiful and delicious!*

    Ground chicken makes a tasty burger. Add onions, poultry seasoning, an egg to bind, coat with whole wheat crumbs and broil. You can also buy frozen chicken patties in health food stores.

- **Turkey** is sometimes a bother, and leftover frozen turkey is not as good as freshly cooked. Have your butcher cut a small hormone and antibiotic-free turkey in half and freezer wrap; when you want turkey, bake a half and eat for lunch and dinner until it's gone. A quick leftover turkey or chicken recipe is:

> Melt 2 tablespoons Better Butter in a skillet and low-heat sauté 1/4 cup or more chopped onion, one chopped garlic clove, and 1-1/2 cups unpeeled diced potato for 15 minutes or until soft. Add 2 cups diced chicken or turkey, 1/2 teaspoon salt, and heat through. Mix in 1 cup or more natural canned chicken broth and 1 tablespoon minced fresh parsley. Add more chicken broth as needed to keep the hash from being dry.

- **Rabbit** is lower in fat and cholesterol than any other mammal meat, and higher in protein. You can use it in any chicken recipe. Some people are unwilling to try rabbit because the whole pieces "look too much like rabbits." Have your butcher grind rabbit and use it in any hamburger recipe like chili, spaghetti sauce, or rabbitburger. I've yet to look at ground rabbit and see a rabbit! Add sage and salt to ground rabbit for delicious low-fat sausage.

- **Eggs** are capable of producing life, and are a perfect food. Buy hormone and antibiotic-free eggs, from a free ranging flock with a rooster, for best nutritional quality. Cholesterol in eggs is over-rated as a cause of high cholesterol in our blood. Moderation is the key word. Prepare eggs hard-cooked, soft-cooked, poached, baked, or low heat stove set. An opportunity to use your creativity in preparing eggs is a low-heat omelet:

> Wipe a cast iron skillet with sesame oil. Whip 1 tablespoon water and a dash of salt with 2 eggs. Pour into skillet and bake at 350 degrees until set. Place your favorite filling on half the omelet, fold the other half over, and cut in half to serve two. Some foods good in omelets include soy or rice cheese; salsa; bean sprouts; raw green onions; healthy sausage cooked and blotted dry; cooked onion, garlic, or green peppers.

8. DAIRY PRODUCTS

Healthiest milk is non-fat; preferably non-fat soured forms such as yogurt, kefir, and buttermilk. Friendly bugs in yogurt help with digestion, form colonies that manufacture some B vitamins, and push out unwanted bacteria and Candida yeast. Soy yogurt has the same good bacteria.

If you reduce meat, soft drinks and processed foods in your diet, your body's calcium need would most likely be satisfied by non-dairy sources like seeds and nuts, dark green vegetables, fish and seafood, seaweeds, beans, egg yoke, chicken, molasses, carob flour, and occasional non-fat or low-fat dairy or soy products.

> *If you can tolerate "occasional" dairy yogurt, you might try adding a little maple syrup and pecans to plain yogurt; or better yet to vanilla soy yogurt.*

9. NUTS AND SEEDS

> *"Seeds contain nearly every single food element that has been discovered. and doubtless all the additional factors not yet identified. No other one food is so rich in nutrients as the seed, containing as it does the life forces needed to build the new generation. Seeds have highly potent therapeutic values."*
>
> — Dr. Bernard Jensen

Tucked inside every seed is the secret of life. Seeds provide the body with vitamins, minerals, proteins, trace elements, and the right kind of essential fatty acids. Look for every opportunity to use seeds in soups, casseroles, sauces, breads, muffins, waffles, pancakes, salads, salad dressings, blender drinks, and sprinkled on almost anything you can imagine. You may eat a few small fruit seeds from apples and grapes; larger quantities like cantaloupe and watermelon can be blended in any liquid and strained to make a delicious drink. Why should your garbage can be healthier than you are? Dr. Jensen warns that apple seeds from heavily sprayed orchards can contain up to 75 percent of the spray. Organically grown food is always best.

Nuts and seeds should be eaten fresh and raw, except peanuts, which are legumes and must NOT be eaten raw. Commercial oil-roasted nuts and seeds are often prepared in rancid oil at high temperatures, so dry roasted is better; raw is best. A good source for organic nuts and seeds is Walnut Acres (800-433-3998).

Nuts and seeds should be stored in the freezer as they turn rancid quickly. Nuts in the shell should be consumed quickly, or frozen. Nuts will not freeze solid due to the high fat content, and can be eaten right from the freezer. Do not buy broken nuts or products with broken nuts, as they can become rancid before the package is even opened. Rancid oils are hard on the liver; never eat any nut or seed that tastes rancid.

Nuts contain large amounts of high quality protein and beneficial essential fatty acids. They are high in fat, so they should be consumed in small amounts. Eight to ten nuts (or what you can fit in the palm of your hand) at a time are recommended for good digestion. Too much of a good thing doesn't make it better! You can have more after a few hours. Hazelnuts, macadamia nuts, pecans, almonds and pistachios are high in monounsaturated fats. Some people prefer the nut butters, and these should be used up quickly when opened. A favorite lunch or snack is:

> *Put a brown rice cake in the oven at 200 degrees for ten minutes to crisp. Wrap in foil if you are taking it to work. When ready, top with a layer of almond butter or any nut butter available in health food stores, or fresh peanut butter. Top that with banana slices if desired...DELICIOUS!*

Nut or seed milk is a substitute for milk, and can be used in any recipe for superior nutrition. This lacks milk sugar so recipes like muffins, pancakes or waffles need added natural sugar like pure maple syrup to brown. Recipe in *SOURCES OF CALCIUM* in the Internal Energy chapter.

Sprouting seeds improves their nutritive value. Sprouts are the most **ALIVE** food we can put into our bodies, and you don't need a farm to sprout seeds! All you need to become an organic gardener is enthusiasm, and room to set a small pan in the light. Get one of the many fine books available on seed sprouting techniques. You can buy grass seed from pet shops, and sprout to give your indoor cats the grass they love. HAPPY SPROUTING...THE REWARDS ARE TERRIFIC!

10. WATER

Water is the #1 health problem in the world! The true meaning of a preventive approach to health care is to first exclude the simpler causes of disease, and then think of the more complicated. The simple truth is that dehydration can cause any symptom or disease.

Dehydration eventually causes loss of function; various "signals" called symptoms have been considered the indicators of disease. Instead of providing water for these "signals", modern medicine silences them with drugs. **REMEMBER TO FIRST DO NO HARM. CONSUME EIGHT GLASSES OF PURE, FILTERED WATER DAILY** (or one ounce of filtered water for each two pounds of body weight).

City water, even well water in our chemical society contains chemicals the liver must detoxify. Water from *ANY SOURCE* should be put through some purification system. Since you absorb 60 percent of what goes on your skin, a shower or bath can put unwanted chemicals into the body. Showering with chlorine can cause dull, brittle hair; flaky scalp; burning eyes; dry skin; skin rashes; and hot chlorine-filled steam invading your lungs. When chlorine combines with organic matter in water, volatile pollutants like chloroform are formed, which can cause liver and kidney damage, depression, and is a suspected carcinogen. A good defense against poisons in your water is essential fatty acids.

Reverse osmosis or distilled water is recommended over most filters. Many filters do not remove fluoride or parasites. Check your local phone book for reverse osmosis units from Culligan. N.E.E.D.S. catalog has water systems and other environmental products (1-800-634-1380); Doulton Ceramic Water Filter is a good filter (1-800-444-3563, ask for Jan and mention my book for a discount). **Highly recommended:** *YOUR BODY'S MANY CRIES FOR WATER* by F. Batmangheilidj, M.D.

[] [] [] [] []

BREAKFAST OR BRUNCH SUGGESTIONS

The body works in rhythms that allow certain functions to perform best during certain times. It is called Circadian Rhythm and if you acknowledge the cycles, it could have a positive effect on your health:

```
Nutrient Ingestion - Digestion............noon to 8PM
Nutrient Distribution - Utilization - Rest....8PM to 4AM
Waste Elimination...................4AM to noon
```

With all the elements of health stacked against our modern society, it could be beneficial for you to eat light before noon. What you eat is important, so hard-to-digest, high-fat red meat like sausage is not recommended. Small amounts of easy-to-digest foods, especially high fiber foods that jump-start your intestines, liquids, and fresh fruit that gives you energy, are all good choices.

Some suggestions listed may not be perfect food combining, but this book is for people wanting to make healthy changes without alienating the family, or stressing themselves. If you drink a glass of filtered water 1/2 hour before you eat, work on pH balance and other digestion principles discussed in the Digestion chapter, you will digest *"healthy"* food better. Some people who are very ill may need to follow stricter food combining rules; some people are more motivated than others to follow perfect recommendations. For the majority reading this book, these suggestions will be a helpful place to start:

1. Whole wheat waffles or pancakes from recipe provided can be made in double batches and leftovers frozen. Warm, and top with maple syrup, Better Butter, and a few chopped nuts or seeds. For brunch add an organic egg on the side,
2. Cut toasted whole wheat bread into cubes and mix with an organic soft-cooked egg and sea salt.
3. Finger food for rushed mornings can be organic hard-boiled egg, a piece of fresh fruit, a few nuts, or whole grain toast. You can top toast with Better Butter, freshly ground peanut butter, nut butters, or naturally sweetened fruit jams.
4. Stretch your imagination and "create" an omelet.
5. Cut up an orange or a grapefruit and top with a little maple syrup and sunflower seeds; or add water for a blender drink.
6. Scrambled eggs will be much lighter if you beat in 1 tablespoon soy or rice milk for each egg; pinch of seasalt.. Melt 1 teaspoon Better Butter for each egg in pan, and cook eggs on low heat. Serve with whole grain toast.
7. Make your favorite whole grain muffin recipe and freeze. Set several muffins out to thaw before you go to bed; 30 seconds in the microwave the next morning gets you going. Add a piece of fresh fruit. Instead of muffins make this excellent zucchini bread:

> *Cream 1/2 cup butter and 1/2 cup honey. Beat in 2 large eggs. Add 1 cup grated, packed raw zucchini and 1 teaspoon natural vanilla extract. Add 2 cups whole wheat flour, 2 1/2 teaspoons baking powder, 1 teaspoon ground cinnamon, full 1/2 teaspoon seasalt. Beat well until mixed. Bake in 8 inch square PAM sprayed pan at 350 degree oven for 30-40 minutes.*

8. Leftover mashed or sliced baked potato or brown rice can be low-heat sautéed in a small amount of Better Butter, with or without an egg, and topped with a few seeds or chopped nuts.
9. If your high-energy morning work requires a "hearty" breakfast, you can make your own low-fat sausage with ground hormone and antibiotic-free chicken, turkey, or rabbit, sage to taste, and solar sea salt. Add fresh ground black pepper at the table if you wish, but cooked pepper is hard on the liver. Ground pepper can turn rancid, so always grind whole peppercorns as needed. For brunch you can top sausage patties with sunflower seeds and eat accompanied by #8.
10. Tapioca does not need to be a milk base; for one serving of fruit tapioca soak 1/8 cup Minute Tapioca in 1/2 cup fresh orange juice, 2 teaspoons pure maple syrup (or more based on sweetness of orange), 1/2 cup water, and a dash of salt for 5 minutes. Bring to a boil and simmer 5 minutes; let stand 10 minutes. Eat warm, topped with a few chopped pecans; great for a relaxing weekend morning change.
11. Chill and slice cooked cereal; warm on low heat in Better Butter, and top with chopped nuts or seeds. Tastes good with soft-cooked egg or homemade sausage. Recipe is as follows:

> *Mix 1 cup cornmeal with 1/2 cup cold water. Heat 2 cups water with 1/2 teaspoon salt in a double boiler. Stir in cornmeal and cook until thickened, stirring occasionally. Cook covered on very low heat for 20-30 minutes. Pour into a loaf pan and chill. Slice and warm in a little Better Butter, serve topped with a small amount of maple syrup.*

12. Oatmeal, wheat, rye or buckwheat cooked cereal, topped with pure maple syrup, finely chopped almonds or pecans, and rice

or soy milk. Health food stores carry some nutritious, chemical free dry cereal that is delicious with maple syrup and vanilla rice milk.

[] [] [] [] [] []

LUNCH SUGGESTIONS

1. Whole wheat tortillas with heated vegetarian chili (canned or homemade), sprouts, and shredded soy or rice cheese may be rolled up burrito-style.
2. Small baked white or sweet potatoes are delicious topped with a little Better Butter and a few nuts or seeds.
3. Make enough homemade soup to freeze 3-4 quarts; thaw for lunches. I have a "soup making" day, two times a year, and make three different recipes that day. It is a real project, but the rewards are great with a freezer stocked for months. Here is an easy one I make in the oven:

   Butter bean soup: put 1 package navy beans soaked per routine, in 2 quarts filtered water, 2 LARGE chopped onions, 4 LARGE carrots, and 3 teaspoons seasalt in a large oven proof container. Bake at 325 degrees for 3 hours or until tender; add 4 tablespoons Better Butter.

4. Leftover turkey or chicken make great cold salads.
5. Unsalted, natural corn chips can be topped with fresh salsa, chopped green onions, and soy or rice cheese melted on top for healthy *nachos*.
6. Smoked fresh fish (carried in fish markets or health food stores) with whole grain crackers.
7. Vegetarian eggrolls, whole wheat chicken pies, natural chicken or turkey hot dogs and lunch meats are available at health food stores.
8. An all natural hot dog, some sprouts, and fresh salsa on a whole wheat roll is a substantial lunch. Make your own hot dog sauce with natural catsup, cold-pressed mayonnaise, natural mustard, and naturally sweetened pickle relish. If you cannot eat wheat, spread sauce on a large romaine lettuce leaf and fold around your hot dog.

9. Soy or rice milk cheese may be melted on a whole wheat tortilla, topped with chopped scallions, tomatoes, sprouts, green peppers, and sunflower seeds and served immediately.
10. A squash cut in half (butternut is delicious in this recipe), salted lightly, poked all over with a fork and spread with a few teaspoons of melted Better Butter is great for lunch or dinner. Bake for one hour at 350 degrees, basting occasionally with the butter. Top with sunflower seeds.
11. Once a week cook a few baked potatoes, sweet potatoes, and a butternut squash cut in half, all at the same time. Put into refrigerator containers, and when you want a hot, quick snack, heat a serving with Better Butter. You could sauté an egg, or eat fish or chicken with either the white or sweet potato. This sweet potato biscuit recipe is delicious, and easy to make with your stored cooked sweet potatoes:

> *Blend 1 cup whole wheat flour, 1/4 cup dark brown sugar, 1 tablespoon baking powder, and 3/4 teaspoon seasalt. Cut in 1/4 cup butter until mixture consistency of corn meal. Add 1 cup mashed cooked sweet potato, and 1/8 cup rice or soy milk; mix to form a soft dough. Turn out on a lightly floured board, and knead gently for 10 seconds. Roll to 1/2 inch thickness; cut biscuits with a 2 inch biscuit cutter, or use the top of a glass.. Bake about 14 minutes on a PAM coated cookie sheet, 450 degrees.*

12. Chopped scallions and an egg added to shredded zucchini, lightly salted, and coated with whole wheat flour makes a tasty pancake. Sprinkle with paprika and sauté at medium heat in a little sesame oil. You can make extra of these at dinner, and heat at lunch. Top with organic unsweetened applesauce.
13. A good tofu cookbook is a helpful addition to your home library. One of my favorites is a tofu Reuben sandwich:

> *Spread two slices of whole grain rye bread generously with your favorite salad dressing. Sauté 2 slices of tofu 1/2 inch thick in Better Butter, and place on bread. Top with soy or rice cheese; broil until melted. Top with heated sauerkraut and dashes of soy sauce. Top with the second piece of bread and ENJOY . . . DELICIOUS!*

14. Add 1 tablespoon Better Butter and 1/4 cup water to a medium peeled, 1/2 inch sliced eggplant, a medium chopped onion, and 2 chopped garlic cloves in a skillet. Lightly sprinkle with seasalt, and steam 15 minutes on each side, or until soft. Top with fresh pesto sauce (not packaged) you can buy in health food and specialty stores. Serve topped with raw sunflower seeds. This is *great* for lunch or a light dinner. Pesto sauce will keep for several weeks in the refrigerator and can be used to perk up many recipes.
15. The best lunch is to start drinking your blender drink. . .read on!

[] [] [] [] [] []

SPIRULINA - VEGETABLE DRINK

A SUPER FOOD quart blender drink containing the best vitamins, minerals, protein, and supplements to give you energy and keep you nourished for hours. Some combinations may not have taste appeal for you, and others are delicious; keep a record of your experimental results until you become familiar with your favorites. The following are guidelines:

BASE LIQUID:
- 1 cup unchlorinated, unfluoridated water.
- 1 cup soy milk, rice milk or any non-dairy milk.
- 1 cup of any health food store brand of vegetable juice, or natural lemonade.

SUPPLEMENTS:
All supplements should be started at lowest dose, and increased to recommended dose as tolerated:

- 1 tablespoon of Spirulina powder; recommended Spirulina is from Light Force. *(Become a member for $15.00/year and get a 25 percent discount. Call 1-800-722-0444 under ID# 9200-10984).* Light Force also sells an excellent product called Excellerate that activates intracellular energy. If you order this product use 2 teaspoons Spirulina powder, and 1 teaspoon Excellerate per quart of blender drink.

- Ester C buffered vitamin C powder up to 3000 milligrams as tolerated. You should take your maximum dose of Vitamin C daily that does not produce gas. Vitamin C should always be buffered if your pH if normal or acidic, and only ascorbic acid if you are too alkaline (this is discussed in the Digestion chapter).

> *To determine your maximum dose, take a 500 milligram tablet every hour until your stomach starts to rumble, stop for that day; on a daily basis, take 500 milligrams less than amount that gave you gas. Put up to 3000 milligrams in powder form in your daily blender drink; take any dose above that in divided doses throughout the day.*

- 1 1/2 Tablespoons cold-pressed Flaxseed oil in the black bottle in refrigerator section of any health food store. Flaxseed oil supplies vital essential fatty acids; also Hemp oil.
- 2 teaspoons olive oil is a super food for the digestive and elimination systems, liver and gallbladder.
- Colloidal or sea trace minerals available in health food stores. Follow package directions; highest dose may be needed until you start to feel better. Trace minerals are critically important as catalysts in cellular activity, and deficiencies can product any physical, emotional, or mental symptom.
- ***OPTIONAL ADDITIONS***: Juice and pulp of 1/2 lemon, Designer Protein powder from health food stores (this could produce mucus for some people), apple pectin powder (great circulatory cleanser), liquid herbal iron (if you have ridges on your nails), one teaspoon sesame tahini or almond butter (for added calcium}, or one tablespoon lecithin granules (to aid fat digestion). Do not add any supplement that makes the drink taste unpleasant. This **IS** a meal substitute and should be enjoyed.

VEGETABLES:

Add small amounts of five-six raw vegetables (organic if available) to blender. Examples: small piece raw beet (or organic powdered beets 1-800-MY-PINES), several sprigs of fresh parsley, leaf of lettuce (darker foods contain more nutrients; romaine lettuce has twice the calcium and iron, eight times Vitamin C, and 10+ times Vitamin A as iceberg lettuce), leaf of chinese cabbage, one-two radishes, one half or one carrot depending on size, one half stalk celery, leaf of kale or other greens, several slices of summer squash or cucumber, slice of turnip or other root vegetable, or **any other vegetable** EXCEPT onions or garlic because of the strong mouth odor they leave. I do not add fresh tomatoes to the natural lemonade base, because it gives me a *taste* change from the tomato vegetable base drink. Too many vegetables will make the drink thick; the amount should equal a *large* salad.

If you have never eaten a certain vegetable, do not know how to prepare it, or do not like or think you do not like the taste of a certain vegetable, the blender drink is a perfect way to consume foods without any single taste dominating. You do not have to know how to prepare any vegetable, only that you wash it, store it in a glass jar or zip-lock bag, and put a small amount in the blender drink. WOW, HOW SIMPLE!!!

ROTATE ALL SELECTIONS! Do **not** buy the same vegetables you bought the last trip to the grocery store. Eating a wide variety of vegetables is easy with the blender drinks. Rotation of vegetables, and all other food, is beneficial for these reasons:

- *Prevention of allergies. You are less likely to develop allergies to foods you do not eat everyday. Some foods may be staples to you, but you are missing a lot of healthy foods when you become dependent on just a few.*

- *Balancing your nutrients. Foods vary in proportions of nutrients; if you tend to eat the same things daily, you may be eating too much of some nutrients, and not enough of others. A limited selection will most likely produce imbalances and deficiencies. BALANCE is an important word to remember.*

- *More interesting diet. Not everyone will make blender drinks with all the unusual vegetables nicely rotated. Some people eat lettuce, tomato and cucumber salads, and when they run out of those vegetables they go out and get more lettuce, tomatoes and cucumbers. Getting stuck in too many routines could represent the same pattern in your daily life, and prevent you from enjoying challenges.*

EXTRA FOOD TO EAT WITH YOUR BLENDER DRINK:

Nuts and seeds, whole grain breads and crackers, soy dairyless yogurt, rice or soy cheese, one piece fresh fruit, or any healthy choice if you are still hungry.

EQUIPMENT - The best is a HEAVY DUTY blender like Osterizer Classic, with stainless steel sides and a high/low switch. Do not buy a blender with multiple speeds because it is harder to keep clean. The Vita-Mix is more expensive (800-VITAMIX) but helpful if you make bread. Blender drinks are better than juicing vegetables because of the retained fiber.

I love my blender drinks on the five working days, sitting on my desk next to a glass of filtered water. The drink allows me to keep a steady pace without ups and downs, and still feel good at the end of the day. People who travel by car can take their quart blender drink and extra food options in a cooler, any day or everyday. It sure beats a fast food stop for meals. . .and questionable nutrition. On the weekend I have other options that provides a change of pace, so the routine does not get boring.

[] [] [] [] [] []

HELP FOR SHOPPING

1. Read labels on everything you buy and look for hidden sources of sugars, refined flour, and chemical additives.
2. Check your cupboard for canned goods, and evaluate whether these products could be purchased fresh, lower sodium levels, less chemical additives, lower fat, and lower sugar. Some products like tuna or sardines can be purchased in the grocery store, but products like vegetarian chili, tomato sauce, chicken broth, soup, and beans may be best purchased from a health food store. Grocery stores are starting natural food sections, so more things will be available there.

3. Purchase a recipe file box for your favorite healthy food recipes. Keep only family favorites of recipes that do not have the best health ingredients, and discard the rest.
4. Eliminate purchases of new foods containing:

Artificial color	Refined flour	Sodium Nitrate
Artificial flavoring	Monosodium glutamate	BHA
Refined sugar	Sodium Nitrite	BHT

5. Purchase a pressure cooker for quick nutritious meals.
6. Collect large glass jars to store washed vegetables in refrigerator.
7. Purchase a heavy-duty blender if you do not have one. It is an investment in your future.
8. Replace aluminum cookware with stainless steel, Corningware, or iron. Buy aluminum-free baking powder.
9. Get a filter for your well or city drinking water and a shower filter for city water.
10. Purchase cookbooks geared to more healthy eating; especially reducing sugar, fat, red meat and dairy products.
11. Put a "To Buy" shopping notepaper on your refrigerator door so you can jot down special needs as you remember.
12. Purchase cold-pressed oils high in monounsaturated fat like flaxseed, olive, almond, avocado, canola or peanut. Keep refrigerated after opening.
13. Purchase an assortment of nuts and seeds to eat as snacks or use in meal planning.
14. Purchase natural sugars like honey, maple syrup, and molasses. Also have on hand a small supply of better sugars for those special needs like Sucanat, fructose, or Stevia.
15. Purchase whole wheat, spelt flour, brown rice, and other grains; keep all grains in the refrigerator.
16. Purchase a healthier version of stock food supplies from the health food store such as catsup, mayonnaise, mustard, relish, salsa, chicken stock, tomato soup, and sea salt, to mention only a few. This turnover may need to be gradual because of finances, but you do have purchasing power on new items.

[] [] [] [] []

So, you want to feel good, and enjoy life. Good nutrition is the best place to start. The first stage of deficiency begins when you mishandle food, make poor selections, fail to digest your food, or fail to utilize your digested food. You live or die on a cellular basis; when the supply of nutrients stops, your needs are drawn from your reserves. If the nutrients are not available, your body shows signs of stress with symptoms like indigestion, irritability and depression. If you are treated symptomatically, as I was, you keep getting sicker.

I've just touched the surface with the information available on the subject of nutrition. This is a LIFETIME study, and the more books and newsletters you obtain, the more knowledgeable you will become. I have listed my favorite resources in the back of this book. When you rely on social pressures, advertisements, and family habits to "inform" you on facts that affect your well being, you may be unhappy with the direction of your health. Assuming responsibility for your health means YOU become aware of what it takes to allow the body to work at optimum performance or heal itself.

We love to blame our poor health on heredity, but the influence of heredity is minimal compared to nutrition. The basic condition that makes our cells vulnerable to disease is inadequate nutrition. When the nutritional balance of the body is restored, symptoms tend to disappear.

Diet is what you put into your mouth; nutrition is what your cells actually receive. That means good digestion. . .so read on. . .

CHAPTER 3

DIGESTION

YOU EAT TO LIVE. . .NOT LIVE TO EAT. YOU LIVE OR DIE ON A CELLULAR BASIS, AND WHAT YOU EAT DETERMINES CELLULAR HEALTH. YOU DERIVE NO VALUE FROM FOODS THAT ARE NOT DIGESTED.

Of the three major life-sustaining nutrients. . .protein, carbohydrates, and fat. . .the chemical structures of protein are the most fundamental. Proteins alone serve as the building blocks out of which all the cells of our bodies are constructed; the other two factors are used principally as energy sources. Without protein, the human body would not exist.

Proteins, carbohydrates, and fats ingested as meat, bread, fruit, or other food are not usable by the body in that form. Changes that happen to food as it is affected by different enzymes, refine the food into nutrients that can be used by the cells.

This process of disintegrating and refining of food is called DIGESTION. It is partly mechanical as in chewing, swallowing, and churning of foods. It is also partly the changes foods undergo as they are affected by proteins known as enzymes. The basic process of digestion is the splitting of a compound into fragments by enzymes specific for each type of food; and each enzyme has well-defined limitations.

IT IS POSSIBLE THAT EVERY KNOWN DEGENERATIVE DISEASE MAY HAVE ITS ORIGIN IN ENZYME DEFICIENCY. It is estimated that the human body requires about 600 various enzymes to maintain proper health. **COOKING DESTROYS ALL NATURAL ENZYMES, AND REQUIRES THE BODY TO PROVIDE ALL THE ELEMENTS OF DIGESTION.**

[] [] [] [] [] []

A WALK THROUGH THE DIGESTIVE PROCESS

Taking the journey with our food, from the time it enters the mouth to the last stage of digestion, is a fascinating story from beginning to end. The digestive process changes carbohydrates to simple sugars called monosaccharides, proteins to amino acids, and fats to fatty acids. It all begins with your first bite of food.

CARBOHYDRATES

Carbohydrates start digesting in the mouth. The three major sources of carbohydrates in the human diet are:

1. *Sucrose - refined sugar*
2. *Lactose - milk sugar*
3. *Starches - complex carbohydrates present in many foods like white potatoes, sweet potatoes, beans, and grains*

Only **starch** digestion begins in the **alkaline** mouth from the **ptyalin** enzyme in the saliva. The quality of this process can be affected by the combinations of food you eat. An acid food eaten with a starch can change the mouth to *ACIDIC*, and prevent the ptyalin from starting starch digestion in the mouth.

You can experience the digestive effect of ptyalin by chewing bread for several minutes. It becomes sweet from the liberation of sugars.

The action of ptyalin continues in the stomach until the food is completely mixed with gastric juices, which are acidic. Starch digestion stops at this time, and completes the process in the *ALKALINE* small intestine. Before starches enters the liver, they are simple sugars called monosaccharides.

PROTEINS

Proteins are fragmented in the digestive tract into complex chains of amino acids. Just like the composition of a word from our alphabet letters, amino acids (the letters) at the cellular level begin to form new proteins (the words) which become new cells in the body. As the omission of even a single alphabet letter prevents the completion of a word, so does a deficiency of a single amino acid inhibit the proper formation of these chemical structures into new proteins. The new proteins are used for cellular reconstruction.

There are basically 22 amino acids. All are "essential" but the following must be obtained from your diet: arginine, histidine, isoleucine, leucine, lysine, methionine, phynylalanine, threonine, tryptophan, and valine. These may not be meaningful to you, but if you run across them in articles you should know they are not vitamins, enzymes, or something else. The essential amino acids cannot be made by the body, and nothing can substitute for them.

If there is a deficiency of one or more amino acids, the protein changes do not occur at all, or occur in proportion to the insufficiency of some amino acids. These tremendous variations in amino acid chain-like structures are partially responsible for the ability of one individual to eat a particular food without ill effects, while another person encounters severe allergic reactions.

PROPER DIGESTION CAN IMPROVE ALLERGIC REACTIONS!

The digestion of proteins starts in the stomach. The protein enzymes in the stomach are active only in an acid medium. Gastric glands secrete a large amount of **hydrochloric acid (HCL)**, that activates the protein digestive enzyme **pepsin**. Pepsin splits proteins and begins protein digestion. HCL has two functions:

1. *To promote pepsin activity; HCL deficiency is a frequent cause of allergies.*
2. *To sterilize the stomach contents, called CHYME. A dog can raid a garbage can and not get sick, because he has a lot more HCL than humans.*

Protein breakdown is very complex and many enzymes act in different stages of digestion. No single enzyme digests protein all the way to amino acids, the final stage which is completed in the small intestine. Proteins are split into three forms in the stomach in a time period based on:

- amount of protein in the meal
- size of the chunks of protein
- amount of fat in the meal (1 1/2 - 4 hrs. or longer)

Acid chyme empties into the duodenum (the first part of the small intestine), then is alkalized by sodium bicarbonate from the pancreas. It mixes with intestinal bacteria, enzymes from the pancreas and small intestine to continue the digestion of starches, fats, and proteins. The health of the small intestine is greatly affected by balance in microorganisms, Candida yeast, parasites, pH balance, and water.

The common factor of any symptom of poor digestion, heartburn, stomach distress or inflammation is the change initiated by dehydration. Water means distilled or filtered water; it does not mean regular tea, coffee, alcohol, or manufactured beverages. They contain dehydrating agents and get rid of the water they are dissolved in, plus some from the body.

A preference for soda and juice will reduce the urge to drink water, even when the soda or juice is not available. You end up feeding Candida yeast and parasites. . .and still produce dehydrated cells.

Do not drink in large amounts at one time, thinking you can undo the damage of many months or years of dehydration by excessive intake in a few days. You need to drink a little at a time over the whole day for months, before full hydration of the body is achieved. Symptoms like nausea, or a dislike of water will change as you become more hydrated.

FATS

Essentially, all fat is digested in the small intestine; the first stage is breaking up the fat globules by bile from the gall bladder. The gall bladder does not release bile if you just eat fruit or vegetables, but bile is released when any fat enters the small intestine. If you do not have a gall bladder (it is one of the most performed surgeries in the U.S.), you have bile produced by the liver dripping continuously into the small intestine.

Some digestion of fat occurs from the small intestinal enzymes and healthy bacteria, but the most important action is from the pancreatic enzyme **lipase**. Fats are broken down to fatty acids and glycerol before entering the blood to go to the liver.

Most absorption of nutrients occurs in the small intestine, as well as forming some vitamins like K, B1, B2, B12. The job of the entire large intestine is to receive the fluid waste products of digestion and store them until they are released from the body.

PANCREAS

Let's take time here to discuss the pancreas, which is responsible for producing digestive enzymes, alkalizing the small intestine, producing insulin to regulate blood sugar levels, and producing a special kind of alcohol (a deficiency can cause cold hands and feet, or general chilliness in all seasons). Stress, alcohol, drugs, sugar, and refined food all over stimulate the pancreas and eventually lead to its inability to produce either the acid-neutralizing bicarbonates or enzymes. The suggestions in this chapter (especially for a healthy liver), the good food discussed in the Nutrition chapter (especially the Spirulina blender drinks), and a parasite kill-off product two or three times a year (parasites can compromise the health of the pancreas), will help protect this valuable organ.

[] [] [] [] [] []

MANY PEOPLE ARE OBLIVIOUS TO THE PROBLEMS OF DIGESTION, BECAUSE THEY THINK OF DIGESTION AS AN AUTOMATIC PROCESS THAT PROCEEDS WITH A CERTAIN DEGREE OF PERFECTION. **MAKING ASSUMPTIONS THAT THE FOOD YOU EAT IS ALWAYS DIGESTED, AND THAT THE DIGESTED FOOD IS ALWAYS ABSORBED, COULD BE THE FIRST WRONG STEP TOWARDS DEGENERATIVE HEALTH.**

We derive no value from undigested food. Undigested food in the digestive tract produces poisons that clog cells and lead to disease. Our society's first reaction is to treat burning sensations, heavy feeling after meals, nausea, vomiting, cramps, intestinal spasms, burping, poor appetite or constant hungry, sleepy after meals, and heartburn with modern medicine's "new and improved" products.

If your day is a continuous picnic, the stomach becomes an overloaded storage tank for undigested food. The outcome of this routine is fermentation, gas, mucus, and alcohol waste products that make you run to the corner drugstore for relief...AGAIN! Public opinion does not consider poor digestive symptoms a serious problem, because we have a wide selection of highly advertised, competitive over-the-counter digestive relief choices. You may feel better, which is the *MOST DANGEROUS* of all because you are unaware of the collective damage of poisonous wastes. Treating only the symptoms, you would probably suffer these symptoms the rest of your life (which could be shortened unnecessarily). Or...you could treat the **CAUSE** of the problem.

*REMEMBER, YOU ARE NOT WHAT YOU EAT,
YOU ARE WHAT YOU DIGEST!!!*

ARE YOU READY TO IMPROVE YOUR DIGESTION?

Some people take strict health suggestions and follow them to the letter. However, many people in this country are too busy living the American dream to do every healthy recommendation all the time. Those who want to be super-strict would find controversy in areas of this book. I am not trying to sway the thinking of those already dedicated. I'm trying to present a starting place for those who never before thought they had to learn about the subject of digestion. For those beginners, here are some guidelines:

1. WHEN SHOULD YOU EAT YOUR PROTEIN AND WHEN SHOULD YOU EAT YOUR SALAD?

There are conflicting opinions; reading can produce total confusion. In Europe, they eat their salad after the meal.

> ***One opinion:*** *Every meal should begin with raw foods because you need enzymes of raw food to help digest other foods.*

Another opinion: Protein foods need lots of HCL for proper digestion in the stomach. If the stomach is first filled with a large salad which does not require HCL for digestion, the protein eaten afterwards may not be digested well because the diluted HCL is not strong enough to activate the protein enzymes.

My recommended opinion: A large salad should be eaten with protein, or after, but best not before protein. Raw foods do activate intestinal enzymes, but the digestion of protein begins in the stomach first.

2. SIMPLE FOOD COMBINING

A strict version of this may need to be considered for people with severe digestive problems, or people recovering from a serious illness who need the best digestion. Correct food combining books best describe this guide to digestion. For most people, some principles discussed are too strict, and contradictory to our American way of eating (like no starchy and acidic foods together, which means no more sandwiches). There are, however, some principles that should be considered by everyone:

- *The simpler the meal, the better chance you have of digesting it.*
- *Fats and proteins are not a good combination. A high-fat diet can inhibit the gastric juices and keep the food in the stomach hours longer, causing some foods to ferment. Eat a low-fat diet, but always remember you NEED essential fatty acids.*
- *Do not eat any form of sugar or sweet fruits with a meal containing normal protein intake (especially hard-to-digest animal protein). Sugar will ferment if delayed in the stomach. The exceptions are RAW pineapple and RAW papaya, which contain protein digesting enzymes. You may have a "special occasion" recipe that does not fit this rule. Both my sons want "strawberry lamb chops" for their birthday dinner. These special occasions are not as important as your DAILY choices.*

- *Desserts at the end of the meal combine poorly with almost every other part of the meal. They only complicate digestion; if you must have dessert, eat it alone one-two hours later.*
- *Fruits and vegetables are best eaten separately due to digestive interference in the same area of digestion.*
- *The rule for fruit is - EAT IT ALONE OR LEAVE IT ALONE! Melons, especially, will decompose quickly if held up in an acidic stomach, and will ferment. Fruit may be used in Spirulina drinks because that vegetable protein is in a nearly digested form.*

3. EATING SMALL MEALS, EATING SLOWLY, DRINKING WATER BEFORE MEALS AND CHEWING FOOD EXTREMELY WELL!

"Drink your solids, and chew your liquids." If you chew well, eat small amounts, drink eight ounces of distilled or filtered water 15-30 minutes before eating to churn food for more effective enzyme action, and have enough HCL, about 98 percent of protein will be digested.

> *You may want to add apple cider vinegar to the water before meals to activate hydrochloric acid, and improve digestion. Suggest you read APPLE CIDER VINEGAR by Paul and Patricia Bragg.*

4. THE "NEVERS":

- Never chew gum on an empty stomach as it fools the body and causes digestive juices to flow. This can cause ulcers, and stomach distress, or other digestive symptoms.

- Never eat if not hungry, feverish, in pain, chilled, or emotionally upset (which greatly affects the digestive process). If you do eat, choose easy-to-digest foods like liquid drinks, raw fruit or vegetables.

- Never drink icy cold, or hot drinks with meals because sudden changes slow down the digestive process. Never drink a lot of liquid throughout the meal; this is not a good time to catch up on your daily intake of water. Take supplements with the water before meals, or with a little water after the meal.

5. PROVIDE A GOOD MEDIUM FOR HEALTHY INTESTINAL BACTERIA.

Foods such as yogurt (soy preferred), or other cultured low-fat milk products (if no milk allergy or mucus symptoms), sauerkraut, soured vegetables, or sour bread, will help grow the healthy bacteria needed for good digestion.

> *Products like Flora Balance, available in health food stores, improve intestinal flora in the stomach and small intestines. If you have taken antibiotics, eaten meat, dairy or poultry containing antibiotics, you should also improve large intestine flora with a bowel flora product available in health food stores.*

The diet you eat determines the bacteria in your intestines. A vegetarian will have bacteria that primarily consume carbohydrates. A high meat diet will produce bacteria that act on undigested protein and produce powerful chemical toxins like phenol; phenol is not neutralized by the liver, but passes unchanged into the bloodstream. A person with chemical sensitivities would be wise to eat little or no red meat.

6. ELIMINATE ALL "REFINED" CARBOHYDRATES SUCH AS SUGAR IN ANY FORM, REFINED CEREALS AND WHITE FLOUR.

Refined foods add to constipation and can interfere with the health of the whole interrelated system of digestion, elimination, liver and gall bladder. It is alright to be sociable, have an occasional treat, or celebrate a special occasion with refined "fun food." However, these foods rob your system of nutrients needed for normal body function, so it's best not to be TOO social.

> *The five worst things you can put into your body, other than straight poison and red meat, according to the herbalist Ed Bashaw, are "THE FIVE WHITES":*

1. Refined white sugar and sugar substitutes
2. Refined white salt
3. Refined white flour
4. Refined white shortening
5. Pasteurized, homogenized white milk

7. REMEMBER THE BODY'S CIRCADIAN RHYTHM.

Nutrient "ingestion" and "digestion" is best from noon to 8 PM.

8. DO NOT TREAT CHRONIC ILLNESS LIKE ACUTE ILLNESS.

We may never know how all the drugs on the market affect our enzymes and digestive process. All drugs, because of their toxicity, induce a stress that interferes with digestion and absorption of nutrients **in some way.**

Find out WHY you are sick and eliminate the cause. *DOCTORS ARE FREQUENTLY CRITICIZED FOR PRESCRIBING DRUGS, BUT DRUGS ARE NOT PRESCRIBED FOR PEOPLE WHO ARE HEALTHY!* Consider less traumatic ways to deal with symptoms, such as herbs, whole food supplements, environmental protection with antioxidants, homeopathy, water, and improved nutrition. Living by the following EIGHT LAWS OF WELLNESS may keep you healthy so you do not experience chronic illness.

> *(1) WATER: Drink eight glasses of distilled or filtered water per day (or one ounce per two pounds of body weight). If you have cold/flu or pain symptoms, drink 10 glasses of water for two days.*
>
> *(2) TRACE MINERALS: Unless you eat only organic fruits and vegetables, you need a trace mineral supplement. Take 1 teaspoon colloidal or ionic liquid minerals daily, as lifetime nutritional maintenance.*
>
> *You also need inorganic minerals, available in the Bio-Plasma cell salts, that act as electrical energy in your body (available from health food stores).*

Read THE BIOCHEMIC HANDBOOK by Formur for ways to assist the body to heal itself in acute symptoms; or take three pellets twice a day for lifetime maintenance.

(3) ESSENTIAL FATTY ACIDS: Take two teaspoons Flaxseed oil and one teaspoon olive oil twice a day. Take Flaxseed capsules when you travel, three capsules three times a day. For intolerance to Flaxseed, or desire to rotate, take Black Currant Seed oil or Hemp oil.

(4) pH BALANCE: Test urine and saliva with pH paper a MINIMUM of once a month. Each solution in your body has a proper pH balance; if out of balance, the secretion or solution loses its effectiveness to assimilate or absorb vitamins and minerals. Order DON'T EAT the YELLOW SNOW by Gary Martin, 1-800-321-6917.

(5) CANDIDA YEAST OR PARASITE BALANCE: Recommend a lifetime version of the following diet to control these two disease-producing organisms.

* fresh fruit one time daily only; no fruit juices.
* no refined sugar; keep natural sugars like honey, maple syrup, molasses to a minimum. No milk/dairy (or greatly reduced) due to milk sugar content.
* no **refined** grains except regular pasta no more than once a week if desired.
* ONLY WHOLE GRAINS, combined with starch up to four times a day: whole wheat, oats, rye, barley, spelt, brown rice, corn, millet.
* STARCHY VEGETABLES, combined with grains up to four times a day: all beans, peas, soy, peanut, potato, sweet potato, buckwheat, and squashes.
* Vitamin A increases resistance to tissue penetration by parasitic larvae; eat ample yellow, orange, and dark green vegetables.
* *ALL ANIMAL/FOWL/EGG/FISH/SEAFOOD PROTEIN, OIL/FATS, NUTS/SEEDS, AND ALL VEGETABLES NOT LISTED AS STARCH DO NOT FEED YEAST OR PARASITES.*

(6) ELIMINATION: *Take an HERBAL laxative at bedtime if you do not have a good elimination by noon. Refer to the Elimination chapter recommendations.*

(7) EXERCISE: *Exercise allows the nutrients to get into the cells and the toxic wastes to get out of the cells, at a speed that allows the body to work at optimum performance. EXERCISE and WATER are the two main factors that keep the lymphatic system healthy to eliminate toxic wastes from your body. Oxygen from exercise and deep breathing activates intracellular energy. Your best "health friends" are exercise, water, and oxygen. You should deep breathe five times, six to ten times daily. . .in through your nose and out through your mouth.*

(8) STRESS MANAGEMENT: *Negative energy IS the greatest cause of illness. . .and enthusiasm IS the most important predictor of wellness! Low self-esteem and low self-worth are epidemic in this country, and cellular health depends on the way you deal with stress management. THIS IS THE BOTTOM LINE. HEALTH DEALS WITH ALL LEVELS OF PHYSICAL, EMOTIONAL, MENTAL, AND SPIRITUAL AT THE SAME TIME!*

9. DO NOT DRINK CHLORINATED WATER.

Chlorine destroys intestinal flora needed for good digestion. To eliminate chlorine, let the water set out overnight in a container, or bring to a boil and let it cool on its own. We do not always think of the chlorine in shower water, but you absorb 60 percent of what goes on your skin. Until you get a shower filter, take a short, warm shower with the bathroom door open. Breathing in all that hot, chlorine steam is not healthy. Water (even well water) may also contain other chemicals and micro-organisms that interfere with health; discussed in Nutrition chapter.

10. BE AWARE OF THE TIME RANGE FOR DIGESTION OF DIFFERENT FOODS:

Fruits	*1/2 hour*	
Herbs and vegetables	*1 hour*	
Seeds, nuts, grains	*2 hours*	
Fish	*2 hours*	
Fowl, lamb	*2-3 hours*	*(Heavy protein*
Beef	*3-5 hours*	*is best eaten*
Pork	*5-7+ hours*	*before 6PM)*

[] [] [] [] [] []

SOME SUPPLEMENTS THAT AID DIGESTION

1. **GARLIC** is nature's way of destroying harmful substances, and leaving beneficial organisms to assist in the intestinal digestive process. Garlic is your liver's friend; garlic is very alkalizing.

2. **BEE POLLEN** contains certain enzymes which are essential catalysts in digestion, so pollen is capable of its own digestion, and aids digestion of other foods. It contains up to 30 percent protein, plus essential sugars, vitamins, minerals, and amino acids, all of which in its natural form is a nearly perfect food. As one of the richest foods in nature, it contains every basic ingredient needed to sustain life - A POWERFUL NATURAL SUPPLEMENT.

3. **SPIRULINA PLANKTON** is an algae that contains 70 percent protein, all essential amino acids, highest known source of B12, is a complete food, and an excellent choice of total, natural nutritional protection. SPIRULINA CAN SUPPLY ESSENTIAL NUTRIENTS WHILE THE BODY IS RESTING AND REBUILDING. It is the perfect "multiple vitamin and mineral supplement". The body will always accept natural food better than synthetic fractions of nutrients in a commercial multiple supplement formulated in a chemist's lab. The best "multiple" is not man-made, but all natural *SUPER FOOD* like Spirulina, Blue-Green Algae, Bee Pollen or Barley Green.

4. **BARLEY GREEN** juices are the fast food of the future. . .millions of people are drinking grass for their health. . .not the kind in the yard. Barley Green is a concentrated juice which is dehydrated to a powder at low temperatures, allowing the enzymes to remain alive. There are no indigestible substances. All the nutrients, chlorophyll,

enzymes, vitamins, and minerals are balanced by nature and easily assimilated, being absorbed directly through the cell membranes in the mouth, throat, stomach and intestine.

5. **DIGESTIVE ENZYMES** available in health food stores, lessen the enzyme burden on your body until your body becomes healthier; your goal should always be to balance the body so it functions correctly. Enzymes are not destroyed during digestive chemical reactions, but they do break down and wear out. You can deplete your enzyme potential by living your life at a fast hectic pace. Since our lifestyles are often more stressful than we would like, it may be helpful to temporarily assist your body in enzyme activity, if your urine or saliva pH is not normal.

6. **HYDROCHLORIC ACID** tablets should be taken if saliva pH is too alkaline. Start out with one tablet; add one extra tablet each meal until you feel warmth in your stomach. Next meal take the number of tablets that did not produce symptoms. After reading the Braggs' Apple Cider Vinegar book, you may consider apple cider vinegar before meals to stimulate stomach digestive juices.

7. **MINERALS** are important catalysts in the utilization of proteins, fats and carbohydrates. Potassium is the mineral that opens up a tight digestive system. Any anti-aging program should consider a magnesium/potassium aspartate supplement. The humble prune is a powerhouse of potassium. Plumped with boiling water, they scrub your intestines. All diets should include mineral supplementation, since our foods today tend to be mineral deficient.

8. **B VITAMINS** are easily destroyed by the environment; in physical, emotional, and mental stress; and in processing or preparation of foods. B vitamins affect energy, digestion, nerves, growth, glandular output, emotions, circulation, immunity, and coordination. DO YOU GET THE MESSAGE? THIS IS NO TIME FOR REFINED, OVERCOOKED, AND PROCESSED FOODS!!! Add natural supplements like Bee Pollen and Light Force Spirulina Stress Pack (best B complex I've tested in my practice) to supplement your diet.

9. **ESSENTIAL FATTY ACIDS** in cold-pressed oils, whole grains, nuts, seeds, and legumes, break down to produce chemical

prostaglandins that act as catalysts in body functions including digestion. DON'T FORGET YOUR FLAXSEED OIL.

10. **CAYENNE PEPPER** is a miracle food. It improves circulation and digestion, and is alkalizing. Health food stores carry cayenne in therapeutic higher "heat" units than cooking cayenne; always take with food.

[] [] [] [] [] []

JUICES THAT AID DIGESTION

FRESH, RAW FRUIT JUICES especially lemon, apple, and grape are the cleansers of the human body. In chronic digestive problems, repeated one-day juice fasts can help by giving the digestive organs time to rest and regenerate; more on this in the Elimination chapter. Any tree-ripened fruit eaten fresh is a boost for the digestive system.

VEGETABLE JUICES are the regenerators and builders of the body. They contain **all the substances** needed for nourishing the body, providing the juices are **raw, fresh and without preservatives.** The best vegetables for the intestines are carrots, celery, cabbage, onion, garlic and parsley.

[] [] [] [] [] []

HERBS FOR DIGESTION

THE BASIC ASSUMPTION BEHIND NATURAL HEALING IS THAT THE HUMAN BODY IS LINKED TO THE PROPERTIES OF NATURAL ORGANIC SUBSTANCES. Herbal remedies neutralize or eliminate from your body the harmful substances that impair its power to heal itself. You may not get a dramatic change, but herbs gradually improve health as they influence the system to perform better. *Herbs:*

- *feed, regulate, and cleanse the body naturally.*
- *give the body raw materials to do its own healing.*
- *are not as potentially dangerous as stronger drugs.*
- *should be part of any program in self-responsibility.*

Looking back over the twentieth century there has been a revival of herbalism and natural healing, as the dangers in losing thousands of years of accumulated knowledge have become apparent. The twentieth century's rush for faster, more efficient, more convenient ways to do things has forgotten old ways. This rush from nature has been termed "progress". Physicians have largely turned their medicine over to drug companies with their money-making patents, and this takes the knowledge, and responsibility of SELF-HEALTH away from the individual.

POINTS TO REMEMBER WHEN TAKING HERBS:

1. They frequently accelerate the action of each other, so the most effective way is to take them in combination.
2. Herbs are best taken WITH meals to prevent stomach upset.
3. Herbs are grown wild and contain maximum energy from sunlight and natural growth, providing valuable vitamins and minerals to supplement nutrition.
4. Herbs are dried so they do contain mold for the mold sensitive; it could explain not feeling good on them.
5. Not all herbs are safe. Many contain powerful drug agents that have been used by medical doctors for years (i.e. digitalis). The average herb user is untrained, and habitual use can develop dangerous side effects (i.e. Ginseng Abuse Syndrome, which excites the nervous system). Herbal products are not labeled with side effects like drugs, so you should purchase a good herbal resource book. ROTATION is recommended after two - three bottles, both for possible side effects, and getting the benefits from a variety of excellent herbal choices.

DIGESTIVE HERBS TO DRINK - ginseng, peppermint/other mints, anise, chamomile, licorice root, comfrey (not regularly), fenugreek, ginger root, fennel seed, papaya, cardamon. Sipping room temperature digestive herbs with meals helps digestion.

DIGESTIVE HERBS FOR COOKING - thyme, rosemary, ginger root, papaya, garlic, dill, parsley, cayenne, sage, caraway, fennel seed.

DIGESTIVE HERBS FOR SUPPLEMENTS - saw palmetto berries, catnip, slippery elm, goldenseal, myrrh gum, alfalfa (contains eight essential digestive enzymes - do not use if you are too alkaline).

[] [] [] [] [] []

ACID-ALKALINE pH BALANCE

The Chinese knew about this 5,000 years ago, and called it yin-yang, or the balance of the life force. Modern medicine has almost forgotten it, and our society is paying an unnecessary toll for this lack of awareness.

Man's nature is governed by bio-electrical energy, which pulses as tides from acidity to alkalinity. You are most alkaline during rest, and the acid tide should dominate during the day. For proper body functions, a particular acid-alkaline balance must be maintained. This balance is the regulation of hydrogen ion concentration in the body fluids:

- *Hydrogen is an odorless, tasteless, colorless gas found in all organic compounds.*

- *pH stands for the potential (p) of the solution to attract Hydrogen ions (H); a pH of 7 is always neutral.*

- *a pH below 7 means high hydrogen ion concentration producing a too-acid system.*

- *a pH above 7 means low hydrogen ion concentration producing a too-alkaline system.*

In low resistance to chronic illness, alkalinity dominates. The more alkaline your body pH is, the weaker your digestive juices become.

In poor stress management, acidity dominates. An acid body pH means food must pass through the digestive system quickly to keep from burning the walls of the intestine. This means a decrease in absorption time for nutrients, and less energy for you. *If the urine and saliva pH is not normal, it does not matter what illness is present. Giving the illness a name does not correct the pH imbalance.* What does help is getting the pH back to a normal 6.4. This is a critical part of the EIGHT LAWS OF WELLNESS.

FOR HOME TESTING, TEST FOR pH AS FOLLOWS:

Saturate the pH paper with saliva, and another test strip with urine, first thing in the morning before eating or drinking. Do not test pH before 6AM if you get up during the night. Repeat test for three days to confirm results. Normal urine pH should be 6.4 and saliva pH 6.5. Testing paper is available from Martin Health Systems, 800-948-3411, some pharmacies (most expensive), and health food stores may order it for you.

HELP FOR pH

IF URINE OR SALIVA pH IS TOO ACID - 6.2 OR BELOW, CONSIDER THE FOLLOWING:

- *Take a neutral form of Vitamin C like calcium ascorbate, or Ester-C buffered. Do **NOT** take ascorbic acid! If you have an acid pH, you may not properly utilize Vitamin C.*

- *Eat alkaline forming food listed on page 103. Be aware that excess fruits can aggravate Candidiasis and parasites, and also put a stress on your thyroid or pancreas.*

- *Take Cell Salt Natrum Phosphate as directed on bottle; available in most health food stores.*

Health or illness is on the CELLULAR LEVEL. The "biochemic system of medicine" is based primarily on the "cell theory" and is explained in *THE BIOCHEMIC HANDBOOK* by Formur.

The workers of the cell - the 12 cell salts - are the inorganic constituents of the cell. If a deficiency occurs, a condition arises that produces a symptom. This theory of medicine states that every disease that affects the human race is due to a lack of one or more of these cell salts. To correct this disturbance, you need to know what salts are needed for what action. This knowledge comes from chemistry, so the treatment of disease by supplying the needed cell salts is called BIOCHEMISTRY (bio meaning a combining form).

Tissue salts are safe at all times and cannot conflict with other treatments. They are a natural part of your body chemistry. Cell salts replace what your body is missing, and are valuable options to drugs in chronic or temporarily acute conditions. I am not referring to drugs that may be life saving in emergencies.

- *Take two-four digestive enzymes with each meal, depending on the size of the meal, amount of raw food, and fat content.*

- *No smoking.*

- *No caffeine except Green Tea.*

- *Stress increases acidity. Become aware of the stressors in your life. Either accept them, or come up with a game plan to resolve them. Read Chapter 1 again!*

- *Take high chlorophyll supplements like Spirulina, Super Blue Green Algae, and Bee Pollen which provide complete nutrition that act as a balancing element for body chemistry. Also, Alfalfa, Barley Green, chlorophyll (liquid or gel caps), Royal Jelly, or sesame seeds. All these natural food supplements will not produce acidity. Anyone who is too acidic should have a quart of Spirulina/vegetable blender drink daily!!!*

- *Use all natural Celtic Sea Salt to neutralize the system.*

- *Increase exercise because poor blood flow causes carbon dioxide accumulation and decreases pH.*

- *Any acute acidic condition can be neutralized with Arm and Hammer Baking soda, 1/2 teaspoon in eight ounces of filtered or distilled water; repeat in 30 minutes if necessary.*

IF URINE OR SALIVA pH IS TOO ALKALINE - 6.8 OR ABOVE, CONSIDER THE FOLLOWING:

- *Take ascorbic acid for your Vitamin C; switch to a buffered C or Ester-C when pH is 6.5.*

- *Eat acid forming food listed on page 103.*

- *Take hydrochloric acid (HCL) tablets; or Braggs raw, apple cider vinegar with each meal; or digestive enzymes.*

   When acids formed by foods which are not digesting correctly cause heartburn, and belching of acid stomach contents, we think it is an acid stomach condition. Actually, a lack of HCL can cause food to ferment and putrefy, causing unpleasant symptoms. Antacids help temporarily because they neutralize the fermentative acid, and what little hydrochloric acid may be present. This aggravates the condition by making the system even more alkaline. Check saliva pH before taking any antacid product; do not take if saliva pH is above 6.5.

- *Improve elimination if transit time is not 12-18 hours. To test this, eat whole kernel corn, beets, or spinach for dinner. By noon the next day, you should see the corn, red or green color, depending on what you ate. Take herbal supplements as needed, not commercial laxatives.*

- *Take Cell Salt Natrum Muriaticum, according to bottle directions.*

- *Spirulina and Super Blue-Green Algae balance body chemistry, but in SEVERE alkalinity, Bee Pollen may be best because algae is high in chlorophyll.*

The natural ratio in a normal, healthy body is about four parts alkaline to one part acid. This ideal ratio maintained by your diet provides a strong resistance to disease; it is call the **RULE OF 80/20**. This rule means 80 percent of your food should be *alkaline forming*, and 20 percent should be *acid forming*.

ACID AND ALKALINE FOODS

There are two types of acid and alkaline foods. Acid and alkaline food means how much acidity or alkalinity the food contains in nature. Foods react in the body according to digestion, so acid forming or alkaline forming means the changes foods undergo after being digested. What is important to your health is the acid or alkaline FORMING state of foods.

Acid Forming Foods	Alkaline Forming Foods
Eggs	Unrefined salt
Beef	Sprouted grains
Pork	All vegetables
Lamb	Fruits (expect cranberry, plums, prunes, blueberries)
Chicken	
Fish/Seafood	Herbal teas
Milk/all dairy products	Cooking herbs and spices
Goat's milk	All fresh beans
Grains (except millet, Quinoa, Amaranth)	Untreated oils
	Raw apple cider vinegar
Nuts (except almonds)	Sweet brown rice vinegar
Dried beans (except soybean)	Yeast
Peanuts	Raw honey, Sucanat, Brown rice syrup
Processed sugar, artificial sweeteners, maple syrup, molasses	
Alcoholic beverages	
Peanuts	
Coffee, black tea	
Carbonated beverages	

[] [] [] [] [] []

THE BASIC CAUSE OF DISEASE IS AN IMBALANCE IN YOUR BODY CHEMISTRY, which leads to an imbalance in what is called the **Autonomic Nervous System.** This system regulates all the parts of the body you do not control consciously. . .blood, circulation, digestion, and glands.

TWO BRANCHES OF THE AUTONOMIC NERVOUS SYSTEM:

- sympathetic branch, activated by acidity and calcium.
- parasympathetic branch, activated by alkalinity and potassium.

All organs and tissues have both. One branch excites the organ or tissue, and the other branch slows it down; they regulate each other like a gas pedal and a brake pedal.

When the body is working normally, both branches are in balance, and organs function properly because neither branch dominates. *WHEN ONE BRANCH IS DOMINANT THEN THE OTHER BRANCH IS WEAK.*

THE SYMPATHETIC NERVOUS SYSTEM SPEEDS UP THE FUNCTION OF THE:

- *heart*   - *thyroid*   - *ovaries*
- *adrenals*   - *pituitary*   - *testes*

THE PARASYMPATHETIC NERVOUS SYSTEM SPEEDS UP THE FUNCTION OF THE:

- *pancreas*   - *intestines*   - *digestive system*
- *liver*   - *stomach*   - *colon*

One example of what happens when these two systems are imbalanced:

When your parasympathetic system dominates (pH too alkaline), potassium is INCREASED in the cells and calcium LEAVES your cells. Calcium is necessary for cell strength, so the membranes weaken and become too porous. This allows allergens to irritate or even penetrate the cells. The result provokes an allergenic response as the cells produce excess histamine in defense. In an effort to get rid of the excess histamine, the cells discharge it through the weakened cell membrane. This action irritates the connective tissues, and dilates the blood vessels. Fluids leak from both tissues and blood vessels, causing the swelling and inflammation that produce pain and reactions you call allergy symptoms. NOTE: You can reduce the acidity of this reaction with 1/2 teaspoon of baking soda in eight ounces of water.

WITH SO MUCH STRESS IN OUR SOCIETY, MANY PEOPLE PRESSURE THEIR SYMPATHETIC SYSTEM TO EXHAUSTION. THE DOMINANT PARASYMPATHETIC SYSTEM TAKES OVER, AND SERIOUS ILLNESS AND DEGENERATIVE DISEASE CAN DEVELOP. AS IT TOO BECOMES EXHAUSTED, CHRONIC ILLNESS BECOMES A WAY OF LIFE...AND DEATH. We need to stop blaming heredity for our poor health. A person can improve hereditary tendencies living by the EIGHT LAWS OF WELLNESS.

WHAT FACTORS DEPRESS THE SYMPATHETIC SYSTEM?

- **Prolonged stress** over stimulates this system, and will eventually weaken the sympathetic system.

- **Poor calcium metabolism.** Refer to the Internal Energy chapter.

- **Acid forming foods consumed in excess** will over stimulate the system, and eventually weaken it.

- **Too much Vitamin D** can cause an excess of calcium assimilation, so watch the amount of fortified food you eat. This, again, will first over stimulate the system, and then weaken it.

- **Weakened sympathetic nervous system from birth**; we are producing less healthy children than our forefathers.

- **Low exercise** causes carbon dioxide accumulation, decreasing pH.

- **A deficiency in alkaline minerals** such as organic sodium, potassium, calcium, magnesium, manganese, and iron. This is no time for refined and processed foods.

WHAT CAUSES PARASYMPATHETIC DOMINANCE?

- **Excessive amounts** of some common foods like avocado, bananas, grapes, tomatoes, broccoli, beets, cabbage, carrots, celery, garlic, all lettuce, potatoes, beans, peas, green beans, and parsley contain high levels of potassium and can over stimulate this system. **MODERATION AND ROTATION IN ALL FOODS IS RECOMMENDED!**

- **Constipation** produces an alkalizing substance called "guanidine," which in excess can alkalize the cells and cause the parasympathetic system to become dominant. Both a too acid and a too alkaline system will benefit from a cleansing program you'll get in the Elimination chapter.

- **Too much junk food, and poorly digested red meat and dairy**, puts an overload on the kidneys so they are less effective in controlling proper ratios of acid-alkaline.

- **Poor calcium absorption** to stimulate the sympathetic system.

- **Excessive use of antacids**. . .check your pH!

- **Deficiency of chloride ions caused by prolonged salt restricted diet.** *ABNORMAL RESTRICTIVE DIETS WILL NOT MAKE A BALANCED, HEALTHY BODY!*

- **A lack of hydrochloric acid in the stomach**; low zinc levels reduce stimulation of stomach cells to produce HCL.

- **Poor liver function** reduces absorption of Vitamins A and E needed for strong cell membranes. Without strong cell membranes, alkalinity is more likely to occur.

[] [] [] [] [] []

LEARN TO LOVE YOUR LIVER

The "liver" is very aptly called liv-er; without it, life is impossible. The liver almost never feels painful, yet a person with a healthy liver is a rare exception because of:

- bad diet choices typical in our society.
- multiple addictive habits.
- chemicals in our food and our environment.
- less healthy children being born each generation, which means the liver can be overworked at birth.

One cannot live long without their heart, brain, kidney or pancreas, yet it is proper liver function which prevents these organs from becoming diseased. It is the largest single organ of the body, surpassed by none in the importance of its various activities. It has great capacity to regenerate if deterioration is not extensive, and is the only organ that will regenerate itself if part of it is cut away. It is a magnificent piece of creativity, responsible for over 560 tremendously important functions.

Disease is largely due to 2 changes in the body:
- *nutritional deficiencies*
- *toxic build-up*

A poor functioning liver is involved in both of these problems, so the entire body will be affected.

SOME ACTIVITIES PERFORMED BY THE LIVER:

- Chemicals in your food, drugs, and environment pass through the liver and are either converted into forms usable by the body, or detoxified and discharged into the bile.

    *Your responsibility is to minimize chemicals in your food and environment **so the liver does not have to work so hard**. It takes body energy and nutrients BORROWED from normal body functions to eliminate chemicals you could choose not to use, or be exposed to.*

- Enzymes are made in the liver which aid digestion, and supply the raw materials used by organs, glands, and tissues. This is a *BIG JOB*, and yet your liver does it every day of your life. WITHOUT ENZYMES, LIFE WOULD BE IMPOSSIBLE! THE LIVER CANNOT MAKE OVER ONE THOUSAND ENZYMES ON JUNK FOOD!!! "Coca-Cola does a body good?"

- Antibodies to protect against infectious diseases are produced in the liver.

- The clotting factor which keeps you from bleeding to death is an appreciated liver function.

- The building blocks of proteins - amino acids - are converted in the liver into usable nutrients.

- Normal blood glucose concentration is maintained in the liver by taking excess glucose from the blood, storing it as glycogen, and restoring it to the blood as glucose when needed.

- Conversion of carbohydrates and proteins into sugar and fat when they are needed for energy, or eaten in excess.

- Homeothermic imbalance can be caused by an overactive liver producing heat intolerance, or an underactive liver causing intolerance to cold.

- Cholesterol is formed in the liver, of which 80 percent is converted into bile salts. New amounts of bile are formed in the liver to replace the amount lost through elimination.

BILE SALTS HAVE FOUR MAIN FUNCTIONS:

1. They lubricate the intestines to aid in elimination.
2. They emulsify, or break up, the fat globules into minute size.
3. They help in absorption of fatty acids, cholesterol and other lipids from the intestinal tract.
4. They regularize the proper balance between the healthy intestinal bacteria and the unhealthy micro-organisms like parasites or worms. Poor bile acid production creates a disorder in the intestinal flora, causing some species to disappear and others to multiply.

- Lecithin is produced by the liver to dissolve fats within itself or in the bloodstream, supports healthy skin, feeds muscles, and brain.

- Forms urea to remove ammonia from the body fluids. Without it, extreme toxic conditions develop rapidly.

- Excretes bilirubin, which is the end product of hemoglobin decomposition when blood cells have lived out their life; stores iron from which new blood cells are made.

- Stores fat soluble vitamins A, D, E, F and K; also stores iron, copper, some trace minerals and B vitamins.

Iron is stored in the liver and will remain there unless there is enough Vitamin C in the bloodstream, copper in the hemoglobin, Vitamin E in the tissues, essential fatty acids, cobalt and 19 different amino acids. The "Prima Donna" iron particle will collect in the liver with inadequate B6 (which itself needs enough hydrochloric acid to be assimilated). SO MUCH FOR ONE IRON PILL!!! A better way to deal with iron deficiency is to improve your diet, and balance your pH for better absorption of nutrients. If you need extra iron, take liquid herbal iron products from the health food store.

- Inactivates hormones when they are no longer needed. Very important considering the increase in hormone related cancers like breast and prostate cancer.

REDUCED FUNCTIONING IN ANY OF THESE AREAS LEADS TO CONDITIONS THAT CAN DEGENERATE ORGANS, TISSUES, AND NERVOUS CENTERS.

[] [] [] [] [] []

THE LIVER ACTS AS A FILTER FOR THE REMOVAL OF TOXINS AND NUTRIENTS BETWEEN IT AND THE HEART: The liver has a double circulation system, meaning that it receives blood from both the veins (carry blood towards the heart) and the arteries (carry blood away from the heart). If the body had no way of filtering out chemicals or impurities, they would keep circulating indefinitely, causing permanent change and eventually death. Fortunately, we have several systems for removing them as a back-up for the liver. . .intestines, lungs, kidneys, and skin. BUT THE LIVER IS THE GREATEST PURIFIER OF THEM ALL.

PROBLEMS FROM A MALFUNCTIONING LIVER

- **POOR DIGESTION** includes a red nose, chronic or acute nausea, gas, bloating, belching, anal itching due to the irritation from the heat of fermentation, heartburn, chills, fatigue, headache, sleepy after meals, and a general sluggish feeling.

- **POOR ELIMINATION** could be the root of headaches, low back pain, intestinal spasms, cramps, fatigue, or irritability.

- **URINARY PROBLEMS** that cause you to get up at night can be a sign of food allergies, and liver problems are always a part of allergies.

- **ABNORMAL INTESTINAL ORGANISMS** like worms, parasites, or Candida yeast.

- **INTESTINAL INFLAMMATION** like appendicitis, colitis, diverticulitis.

- **STOMACH ULCER** is always preceded by a liver disorder; food allergies need to be evaluated (especially milk and wheat). IT IS VERY IMPORTANT TO EVALUATE WATER INTAKE!

- **MALNUTRITION** develops because food is not properly utilized by the body. It is not enough to take supplements and eat right. The organs involved with the body mechanics for utilization of nutrients must be healthy. *ANY PROBLEM DUE TO A LACK OF NUTRIENTS GOES BACK TO THE LIVER. ONLY HALF THE NORMAL AMOUNT OF BILE IS PRODUCED BY THE UNHEALTHY LIVER CAUSING CHRONIC POOR DIGESTION.* Vitamin C plays a vital role in the production of bile acid.

    OVERWEIGHT OR UNDERWEIGHT is at least partly due to insufficient enzymes to correctly transform and utilize food; or low intracellular energy. You need normal iron levels to carry oxygen, enough Vitamin C to get iron out of the liver, and normal body pH so the liver can make Q10 to activate intracellular energy.

    Overweight can be a sign of dehydration, since the sensation of thirst and hunger are generated simultaneously in the brain. We assume the urge is to need food, when the body may actually be calling for **WATER**. By drinking water before eating, you may find your "hunger" satisfied.

- **ANEMIA** from a malfunctioning liver leading to destruction of red cells, both old and new.

- **DIABETES** can develop from an excess of sugar in the blood and the urine, if the liver cannot handle the sugar coming from the intestines. The pancreas cannot do it's job without enzymes from the liver.

- **SWELLING of legs and ankles** relate to liver function (also kidney and heart which the liver keeps healthy).

- **SKIN DISEASES** produced from toxic substances not neutralized by the liver like acne, rashes, and liver spots. Candida yeast and parasites can cause skin symptoms, and unhealthy liver function is involved with both.

- **GLANDULAR IMBALANCE** at menopause, and during the menstrual period, can be a problem from a malfunctioning liver. The liver is responsible for detoxifying female hormones that produce sore breasts and "change of life" symptoms when they accumulate.

- **NERVOUS SYSTEM DISORDERS** from retained toxic wastes can affect all systems. The liver must keep up with the toxic load in the body. *YOU CAN DO A LOT TO REDUCE TOXIC OVERLOAD BY REDUCING CHEMICAL EXPOSURES, AND MAKING BETTER FOOD CHOICES.*

- **OVERLOADED LYMPHATIC SYSTEM** is caused when the liver can no longer neutralize all the toxins that circulate in the blood. When blood leakage is filtered by the lymph system, organs like the tonsils get overloaded and inflamed. A tonsillectomy will not solve your long-term problems!!!

- **EAR PROBLEMS** can be due to general congestion of the body. Ringing in the ears may need a liver evaluation.

- **SINUS PROBLEMS, HEAD COLDS, AND CHRONIC RESPIRATORY PROBLEMS** are a waste of time to treat symptomatically and not deal with the liver condition. Colds are more prevalent in the winter when the liver is overworked from a heavier diet and less exercise.

- **REDUCED ABSORPTION OF FAT SOLUBLE VITAMINS A, D, E, F, AND K** due to poor bile production. . .remember Vitamin C.

- **MENTAL DISTURBANCES** from toxic accumulations in the liver poisoning the whole body. The brain is 85 percent water; sometimes the health of that area can be improved with **correct water intake alone.**

- **TENDENCY TO HEMORRHAGE** since the liver produces fibrinogen, an aid to blood coagulation.

- **CANCER** always includes poor liver function as part of the problem.

- **STERILITY AND IMPOTENCE** relate to the quality of our hormone production, from the nutrients our bodies receive from the liver.

- **HYPERTENSION** has liver congestion as its most common cause.

> *All the blood in the body flows through the liver, both to pick up nutrients which the liver stores, and for detoxification. If the liver is congested with toxins or chemicals, overridden with fatty degeneration, or has become hardened from alcohol abuse, a back pressure builds up that can be reflected in the whole body circulation as hypertension.*

> *The Resin-Angiotension (RA) system is the pivotal mechanism for restoring body fluid balance. This system is activated when water is diminished, and tightens the vascular system in a way that can be measured and called hypertension.* ***MANY PEOPLE WHO DRINK EIGHT GLASSES OF WATER DAILY AND FOLLOW THE OTHER SEVEN LAWS OF WELLNESS, NO LONGER SUFFER FROM HYPERTENSION.***

- **HEPATITIS, OR LIVER INFLAMMATION** may result from a sick and weak functioning liver, and a suppressed immune system.

THE LIST OF PROBLEMS GOES ON WITH ARTHRITIS, ALLERGIES, ANEMIA, BODY ODOR, AND FATIGUE. MANY SYMPTOMS RESPOND TO LIVER DETOXIFICATION, WATER TO HYDRATE THE BODY, AND DAILY EXERCISE TO MOVE THE LYMPHATICS (discussed in the Internal Energy chapter).

[] [] [] [] [] []

OUR KNOWLEDGE OF THE LIVER MUST BE EXPANDED AS OUR TECHNOLOGICAL AGE AND EXPOSURE TO CHEMICALS, DRUGS, NUTRITIONALLY INFERIOR FOOD, AND ADDICTIVE HABITS CONTINUES TO GROW. Now that you know WHY you should "love your liver", let's talk about ways to protect the health of this hard-working, valuable organ. Besides the recommendations listed, health food store personnel can assist you in selecting homeopathic and herbal products to support liver health. Consult with your attending physician if you question any recommendation due to your medical history.

SOME FOODS THAT ARE BAD FOR THE LIVER:

- **The basic American diet** produces liver damage!!!

- **Regular alcohol consumption** contributes to general toxicity.

- **Rancid oils** are very hard on the liver. Keep cold-pressed oils, whole grain flour or whole grain bread, and nut butters in the refrigerator; coffee, extra whole grain bread loaves, nuts and seeds in the freezer.

- **Red meat and animal fats** leave undigested waste products that are hard for the liver to neutralize; excess protein depletes calcium reserves.

- **Processed, refined, and chemically additive food** provides minimal nutrition, and must be replaced with food that can give the liver nutrients it needs to perform its many functions. A TWINKIE IS NOT GOOD ENOUGH NUTRITION!!!

- **Margarine, processed oils, coffee, refined flour, refined sugar,** all make the liver deal with chemicals and/or acidity, without getting quality nutritional value!!!

- **Pasteurized milk** is poorly digested by adults; any undigested food is hard on the liver.

[] [] [] [] [] []

SOME CHOICES THAT ARE BAD FOR THE LIVER:

- **Excess fatigue**, both physical and mental, produces toxins that may tax the liver beyond endurance.

- **Overcooked food** destroys nutrients and enzymes, requiring the liver to do more work in the digestive process, plus lose valuable assistance from the lost nutrients.

- **Overeating** strains the liver because of the effort to get rid of toxins resulting from poor digestion.

- **Lack of exercise** reduces the lung's and skin's ability to help the liver in the elimination of toxins.

- **Not enough WATER** reduces the lymphatic system and the kidney's ability to help the liver in the elimination of toxins.

- **Constipation** seriously reduces the bowels' ability to help the liver in the elimination of toxins.

- **Ingested or inhaled chemicals** are hard on the liver. New homes or offices, hobbies, and job choices may not be something that you can or want to change. *YOU MUST, HOWEVER, BE AWARE OF THE DAMAGING EFFECT ON YOUR LIVER, AND MAKE EFFORTS TO HELP IT IN THE STRUGGLE, WITH HEALTHY FOOD, WHOLE FOOD SUPPLEMENTS, FILTERED WATER, ANTIOXIDANT SUPPLEMENTS (an excellent brand sold nationally is Twinlab OcuGuard), AND EXERCISE.*

- **Stress, caffeine, tobacco, and social drugs** make the liver produce enormous elements of defense.

- **Prescription drugs** should be for acute situations, life-saving situations, or body functions (like insulin or thyroid). Always find out WHY you have the problem so you can treat the CAUSE and not just the symptoms. When you have chronic problems, **THE NAME OF THE SYMPTOM, THE NAME OF THE DISEASE IS NOT YOUR PROBLEM... YOUR PROBLEM IS WHY DID YOU GET THE SYMPTOM OR DISEASE.** Treating the symptoms will **NEVER** treat the cause!

THE LIVER WORKS VERY HARD FOR YOU, AND WAS NOT INTENDED TO PUT UP WITH SMOKING; EXCESSIVE ALCOHOL; 8-10 POUNDS OF CHEMICALS PER YEAR; SOCIAL AND PRESCRIPTION DRUGS; HIGH SUGAR, HIGH FAT, REFINED AND PROCESSED DEAD FOOD!!! TO OUR GREAT FORTUNE THE LIVER HAS A TREMENDOUS CAPACITY TO RESTORE ITSELF TO NORMAL FUNCTION.

THE FOLLOWING RECOMMENDATIONS WILL HELP YOU IMPROVE THE HEALTH AND PERFORMANCE OF YOUR LIVER:

DIET

The liver, even with the best diet, has a tremendous job to do. Sometimes the liver gets clogged up with body wastes, resulting from over-consumption of the "dead" foods which are continually being eaten. Instead of treating the symptoms of toxic build-up (like a headache), the sensible thing to do is to lighten the work of the liver. This is best done by eating only such foods as can be easily digested, and will have the fewest end wastes to be cleansed from the system. This is called a MUCUSLESS DIET and it **ELIMINATES:**

- *all processed foods, refined sugar and flour*
- *use of refined commercial table salt*
- *eggs*
- *milk and all dairy products*
- *all red meat (beef, pork, lamb, large wild animals like deer)*
- *any grain that is heated over 130 degrees is mucus-forming*

ALLOWED FOODS:

- *all FRESH fruits and vegetables*
- *all fish, seafood, rabbit, hormone and antibiotic-free chicken and turkey*
- *all nuts and seeds (raw or dry roasted)*
- *all cold-pressed oils*
- *all herbs and spices*
- *all natural sugars like honey, molasses, maple sugar*
- *all sprouted or whole grains, such as stone ground whole wheat, oats, rye, barley, spelt, brown rice, corn, and millet. NOTE: Cooked whole grains are mucus-forming, but provide valuable fiber, B vitamins and other nutrients. Unless a person is trying to eliminate a lot of mucus build-up from years of chronic sinus or respiratory problems, whole grains are allowed cooked as desired.*

- organic eggs needed for recipes are allowed, or as an occasional meal. The word is MODERATION.

◊ ◊ ◊ ◊ ◊

1, 2, OR 3 DAY CLEANSING

Dietary and supplement considerations will work better after an initial liver cleansing program. A cleanse for three days is best, but one or two days is better than nothing. Always consume some oil (preferably olive oil) each day on a juice fast to cleanse the gallbladder. If you cannot fast just on the liquid, you may add the following as desired:

> *- a few raw or dry roasted nuts or seeds*
> *- any combination vegetable salad with homemade olive oil, lemon juice and garlic salad dressing*
> *- skinned hormone and antibiotic-free plain white chicken meat*

Apple or grape juice are both good cleansing choices, but may cause a problem if you have a Candida yeast or parasite overgrowth. In modern society, one degree or another of a Candida yeast and/or parasite problem may exist in most people, **so the safest choice is a lemon juice cleanse:**

> *A simple lemon juice cleanse is alternating a tolerated solution of lemon and distilled water, with distilled water for one, two, or three days. Your total combined liquid intake should be equal to one ounce for each two pounds of body weight. Put juice of two to three lemons in half the water; the rest plain distilled water. Eat a mucusless diet.*

Another cleansing recommendation is:

> *Start with 1 teaspoon, increase to 1 tablespoon as tolerated of extra virgin olive oil; a squeeze of fresh lemon juice; 1/4 increasing to 1/2 teaspoon liquid Kyolic brand garlic available in health food stores; and cold-pressed, whole leaf, and 10X concentrate Aloe Vera juice, 1 teaspoon increasing to 1 tablespoon each morning. Maintain "maximum" dose level for two weeks. Only*

water or fresh fruit until noon; all food should be mucusless for one to two months.

[] [] [] [] [] []

A liver cleanse detoxifies, but also should include rebuilding the cells of the liver. Juices are the cleansers of the body, and vegetables are the rebuilders of the body. Along with your cleanse include vegetables:

Four times a day when fruit juice is not consumed, drink an eight ounce glass of any combination FRESH vegetable juice. Use a home juicer, blend a variety of vegetables in a blender, or eat a large salad.

*Beets are a powerful cleanser and the best vegetable for the liver. NEVER DRINK BEET JUICE ALONE, OR IN LARGE QUANTITIES!! Start with 1/2 **small**, peeled raw beet as a part of every vegetable drink, or shredded on a salad; increase to one small beet as tolerated. Other vegetable choices should include celery, cabbage, kale, spinach, cucumbers, lettuce, carrots, tomatoes, or radishes.*

[] [] [] [] [] [].

DURING EACH CLEANSE. . .

- **Take a warm, relaxing bath or shower in the evening** before retiring. Showering is best if you have city water, because you can buy a filter to remove the chlorine. Nature eliminates poisons through the pores of the skin; a back-up system that reduces the stress on the liver, and allows it to heal. It is necessary to keep the skin clean and free of dead skin cells that clog the pores. Use a body brush daily to remove dead skin cells, that are better down your drain than in your bed. Microscopic mites can cause allergic reactions in some people, and they feed off dead skin cells.

- **IT'S VERY IMPORTANT THAT YOU HAVE A GOOD DAILY BOWEL MOVEMENT BEFORE NOON.** If not, consider enemas, colonics, or bedtime herbal laxative formulas to cleanse the system of the impurities loosened by the juices.

- During the cleanse, have **plenty of fresh air, rest, and sunshine if possible.** You may do stretching or any exercise that moves the lymph (discussed in Internal Energy chapter), but energy needs to go to internal cleansing, so strenuous exercise should be avoided until after the cleanse is over.

- **Practice positive affirmations and LAUGH!!** Laughing massages the liver and helps it function better. . .and, makes your day happier!

[] [] [] [] [] []

SOME FOODS THAT ARE GOOD FOR THE LIVER:

- **UNREFINED, COLD-PRESSED OLIVE OIL** IS THE OIL THAT BENEFITS THE LIVER MOST! Use as much as possible.

- **LEMON IS THE BEST FRUIT FOR THE LIVER,** and can replace vinegar in all seasonings. The liver and lemon are natural together. The secret cure for most illnesses associated with a sluggish liver is the simple lemon.

- **BEETS ARE THE BEST VEGETABLE FOR THE LIVER.** *USE BEETS OFTEN!* They can be cooked, but even better shredded raw on salads or in blender drinks.

- **A high fiber breakfast** helps start bile juice flowing to encourage the elimination that removes toxins from the system.

- **Garlic**'s power to detoxify bacteria in the intestines gives the liver a rest. Garlic helps digestion, increases blood circulation through the liver, stimulates bile production, lowers blood fats, and is a general tonic.

- **All fresh berries** are excellent cleansing foods and are one reason why people tend to be healthier during the summer months.

- **Parsley** should never be left to die on a restaurant platter. It stimulates the liver and helps to prevent gas and indigestion.

- **If all foods are eaten in a fresh, unprocessed form, prepared and served as quickly as possible, nutrients that the liver needs will be**

far more available. Supplements are a big temptation when a person does not feel well. However, no pharmaceutical preparation will ever replace the value of fresh food, and specific nutrients from natural sources like Spirulina, Blue-Green Algae, Bee Pollen, Wheat Grass, or Barley Grass.

SOME HERBS THAT ARE GOOD FOR THE LIVER:

- **Milk thistle** has become world famous as a liver protecting herb. Since herbs work best in combination, you should look for a liver formula containing milk thistle (check health food stores, or mail order companys). Herbs to look for, besides those listed, include: artichoke, Cascara Sagrada, Devil's Claw, Dong Quai, Feverfew, Schisandra, Cloves, and Turmeric

- **Alfalfa** contains chlorophyll for blood purification, and is a good source of nutrients the liver needs. Alfalfa contains B vitamins, Vitamin A, and Vitamin C; do not take alfalfa if your pH is too alkaline.

- **Blessed thistle** aids the liver, digestive system, and lymphatic system. Most bitter herbs are good for the liver like dandelion, and golden seal.

- **Ginseng** is a fantastic tonic for the whole body, and *loves* the liver. It gives the liver energy to heal itself.

- **Licorice** will soothe and help heal the liver.

- **Herbal tea** for liver support includes any herb good for digestion, as well as the following:

    * **Rosemary** is one of the most effective remedies for the liver.
    * **Chamomile** has long been known to help the interrelated system of liver/gallbladder by dissolving gallstones.
    * **Sage** purifies the liver.
    * **Thyme** has antiseptic properties.
    * **Ginger root** helps the liver lower cholesterol levels. Keep fresh ginger root in the freezer until needed, then chop about 1/2 inch off a peeled section. Steep in a cup of hot water for 10 minutes, and strain.

GREEN EGGS AND HAM MAY NOT BE WHAT YOU WANT TO EAT, BUT GREEN DRINKS ARE THE WAVE OF THE FUTURE!!! REMEMBER, THE LIVER HAS AN AMAZING CAPACITY TO REGENERATE ITSELF! A complete program for liver renewal can take three months to one year. Why treat symptoms when a healthy liver is really what the body needs. **THE IMPORTANCE OF MAINTAINING A STATE OF OPTIMUM HEALTH IN THE LIVER, CANNOT BE OVER-EMPHASIZED!!!**

[] [] [] [] [] []

Health is not just what you eat, digest, and eliminate properly, it is also what you think! Regenerating the body is a good time to think how **"YOUNG"** you are rather than how old. As your cells regenerate, you are literally a **"NEW"** person. Think of all the newly born cells in your body . . .no matter how many years you have lived, there is new life being produced this instant!!!

Think new thoughts worthy of those new cells, because there is automatic renewal in the world of cells, but not in the renewal of the mind. YOU HAVE TO SEE TO IT THAT YOUR MIND IN RENEWED!!!

THE BODY RENEWS ITSELF ACCORDING TO THE MENTAL ATTITUDE IT HOLDS!

REMEMBER...

HEALTH IS ON ALL LEVELS OF PHYSICAL, EMOTIONAL, MENTAL, AND SPIRITUAL.

[] [] [] [] [] []

Paul Meynell, editor of RESEARCH NUTRITION wrote:

> *The influence of heredity is minimal compared with that of environment. NUTRITION is an environmental factor. Defective nutrition is a major stress. Many reports from many sources*

indicate beyond doubt that acute diseases, organic diseases, and senile degeneration are all cellular diseases. The basic condition which makes cells vulnerable is inadequate nutrition. By training and social tradition, medicine has to do with DISEASE, and not with HEALTH. Health may be considered just another name for established and maintained BODY CHEMICAL BALANCE. When the balance is restored, through proper digestion of food, "symptoms" tend to disappear.

DIET IS WHAT WE EAT; NUTRITION IS WHAT THE CELLS ACTUALLY RECEIVE.

Our society favors the wrong kinds of liquid, overeating, eating of hard-to-digest proteins, eating wrong combinations, or eating under physical and emotional stress. *WE CANNOT TAKE FOR GRANTED THAT THE PRESENT EATING PRACTICES OF CIVILIZED HUMANS ARE NORMAL. INSTEAD OF HEALTH, WHAT HAS BECOME NORMAL IS A SOCIETY OF SICK AND WEAKENED PEOPLE.*

Good digestion is your insurance plan for protecting health. Poor digestion and stress promotes toxicity that leads to disease. . .best read on and learn how to eliminate toxicity. . .

CHAPTER 4

ELIMINATION

"The natural healing force within us is the greatest force in getting well." - **Hippocrates, Father of Medicine**

Information on symptoms arising primarily from intestinal toxemia have filled volumes. Every symptom does not arise from intestinal toxemia, but it is at the root of conditions more often than is suspected.

The basic premise of organic medicine is that the human body is self-curing when it functions properly. Therefore, the duty of the physician is to promote normal function by:

1. Caring for localized, or acute and crisis symptoms.
2. Restoring the body to its general biochemistry by:
   - eliminating excess waste products from the blood and tissues.
   - supplying nutrients to nourish tissue.
   - restoring body harmony between interrelated systems like glandular/nervous, structural/muscular, and digestive/eliminative.
   - promoting mental and emotional tranquillity.

THIS IS HOLISTIC MEDICINE!

Unfortunately, modern medicine deals more with crisis medicine rather than restoring whole body health. Since modern medicine too often does not resolve the "cause" of the problem, **negative thoughts, body toxicity, cellular dehydration, and disharmony in the whole body continue to produce another crisis.**

"THERE IS ONLY ONE BASIC DISEASE - TOXEMIA, WHICH IS CELLULAR CONTAMINATION."
- Dr. Kurt Donsbach (a noted herbalist)

In most all cases of cellular malnutrition and decreased cellular health, you must FIRST have cellular contamination.

A HEALTHY HUMAN BEING HAS THOUSANDS OF WAYS TO DECREASE CELLULAR HEALTH:

1. Physical shock from serious acute illness or injury.
2. Emotional shock from loss of a loved one, family crisis, loss of financial stability, or serious change in general health.
3. Overeating, since the modern humans inclination is to resist the LAWS OF HEALTH; however, it is alright because we have Alka-Seltzer.
4. Undereating from depression, shock, anorexia, hopelessness.
5. Worry is a comfortable place when low self esteem prevents *action*.
6. Tension produces continued disharmony because *I can't be happy, and life is hard.*

These all interfere with digestion, elimination, absorption of nutrients, and put stress on the lymphatic system (discussed in the Internal Energy chapter). This sets the stage for the gradual accumulation of toxins. These toxic poisons are composed of:

- retained waste products not properly eliminated.
- toxic substances not detoxified by the liver or lymph system.
- absorbed toxic products of abnormal digestion.
- inhaled environmental chemicals, and ingested chemicals.

THESE OVERABUNDANT WASTES SO TYPICAL IN OUR MODERN SOCIETY, DERAIL THE BLOODSTREAM'S DELIVERY TRAIN SO YOUR CELLS DON'T GET WHAT THEY NEED. . . PRODUCING CELLULAR MALNUTRITION.

[] [] [] [] [] []

THERE ARE FIVE THINGS THAT CAUSE SUB-HEALTH CONDITIONS:

1. Congenital deformity
2. Hereditary weakness
3. Organic injury
4. Cellular contamination
5. Nutritional deficiency

The first three represent five percent of all sub-health conditions. *THE LAST TWO REPRESENT 95 PERCENT OF ALL SUB-HEALTH CONDITIONS... AND YOU ARE RESPONSIBLE FOR BOTH.*

One of the most unrecognized sub-health conditions is *parasites*. While Candidiasis has been named the "Twentieth Century Disease", parasites are the unrecognized "All Time Disease" promoters of the past, present and future.

We think Americans are too clean, too civilized, too well fed, and too well educated for parasites to be a serious problem . . . WRONG!!! *PARASITES KNOW NO NATIONAL BOUNDARIES, ARE OBLIVIOUS TO YOUR INCOME, YOUR NATIONALITY, YOUR AGE, AND YOUR BELIEFS.*

More than 80 percent of the world's population is infected with parasites which can range from microscopic to 20 feet long. According to the Center for Disease Control, virtually every known parasitic disease has been diagnosed in the United States. Dr. Hulda Clark in her book, *THE CURE FOR ALL DISEASES*, describes parasites as the cause of both common and extraordinary diseases. She says, "No matter how long and confusing is the list of symptoms a person has, I am sure to find only two things wrong: they have in them pollutants and/or parasites."

Symptoms of parasitic infections run a full range. All parasites weaken your immune system and invite serious illness and degenerative diseases, including that "not well" feeling. Since parasites disturb the balance in the intestines, many effects are digestive symptoms, gas, constipation, diarrhea, bad breath and irritable bowel syndrome. Indirect symptoms that are a result of intestinal disturbance include joint and muscle pains (fibromyalgia syndrome), anemia, allergies, skin problems, nervousness, depression, sleep disturbances, fatigue, and sugar cravings. PARASITES SHOULD BE SUSPECTED IF OTHER FORMS OF TREATMENT FOR GENERAL SYMPTOMS DO NOT HELP!

YOU CAN GET PARASITES FROM:

- inhaling dust containing organisms
- shaking hands with an infected person; or sharing drinks
- playing with your pet; being licked by pets

- from your children who pick them up from friends at school
- from eating raw, unwashed vegetables (salad bars are big offenders)
- raw, rare and undercooked meat and fish and seafood
- restaurant food handlers
- intimate sexual contact; kissing (even on the cheek)
- international, social, or military travel
- rural and urban water systems
- careless diapering in day care centers
- weakened intestinal flora after antibiotics and immune suppressing drugs
- imbalanced bowel flora from low bile acid production

A MAJOR CONTRIBUTING FACTOR TO PARASITE OVERGROWTH IS A COLON CLOGGED AND IMPACTED, WHICH PROVIDES A WARM AND WELL-FED BREEDING GROUND FOR THE EGGS OF WORMS AND OTHER PARASITES TO PROLIFERATE. THEY LOVE CONSTIPATION!!! A HEALTHY INTESTINE STARTS IN THE LIVER.

NATURAL PARASITE TREATMENTS

When you take any product you should expect some symptoms of die-off. These symptoms can be any flu-like symptoms. It is best to take an herbal laxative formula for three days before any parasite product, to flush out any build-up of old fecal material. The parasites lay eggs in that environment. If you do not kill the eggs, you will continue to have new generations of parasites. Some parasite treatment programs are:

- Green hulls of Black Walnut and Wormwood which are the best herbs to kill parasites; cloves are the best to kill parasite eggs. Health food stores carry products containing these herbs.
- Other herbs you should look for in products are pink root, male fern, senna, fennel, Egyptian thorn, and pumpkin seed.
- Garlic, one capsule a day for prevention; two-three daily to treat.
- Colonics just to clean out the colon, but NOT on a regular basis as colonics also flush out good bacteria.
- Products and cleanses that improve liver function are very important since bile acid produced by the liver balances bowel flora so parasites do not want to live there.

- Diet is important since both simple and complex carbohydrates feed parasites.

RECOMMENDED DIETARY GUIDELINES:

FOODS TO ELIMINATE OR RESTRICT:

- Fresh fruit once, no more than twice a day; no fruit juices.
- No refined sugar; keep natural sugars like honey, maple syrup, and molasses to a minimum.
- No milk or dairy due to milk sugar content; reserve dairy for social occasions only.
- No refined grains except social or occasional regular pasta. Whole grain pastas are available in health food stores.

FOODS TO EAT IN MODERATION:

Whole grains and starches break down to simple sugar slowly, and feed parasites (and Candida yeast) less than sugars, fruit, dairy, and refined grains:

- Whole grains include whole wheat, oats, whole rye, barley, spelt, brown rice, corn, and millet.
- Starchy vegetables include beans, peas, soy, peanut, potato, sweet potato, buckwheat, and squashes.

FOODS THAT DO NOT FEED PARASITES OR CANDIDA YEAST:

- Animal/fowl/egg/fish/seafood protein
- Oil/fats
- Nuts/seeds
- All vegetables not listed as a starch. Eat yellow, orange, and dark green vegetables because Vitamin A increases resistance to tissue penetration by parasite larvae.

GUIDELINES FOR PARASITE CONTROL:

- Filter all drinking water regardless of the source, or drink distilled water. Do not purchase any water system without

making sure it removes parasites. Refer to Nutrition chapter for recommendations.
- Wash all foods thoroughly. It is optional to bathe them in 1/2 teaspoon Clorox to one gallon water for ten minutes, or one ounce 3 percent hydrogen peroxide to one pint of water for ten minutes, and rinse well (especially chicken, fish, and meat). I wash my fruit and vegetables in a solution of Shaklee Basic-H. If eggs are soiled, wash well and dry before breaking them open.
- Eat out as little as possible; food handling is a good source of parasites in most restaurants. If your lifestyle requires you to eat out often, it is more important than ever to take a product to kill off a few parasites two or three times a year.
- Deworm your animals twice a year.
- Make sure children who play outside wash their hands, and scrub under their fingernails before eating.
- Wear gloves when cleaning up animal waste.

****Periodic detoxification and cleansing is a must for optimum control. You are NEVER completely free of parasites. **Always** include parasite products during your regular body Spring and Fall *housecleaning*.

[] [] [] [] [] []

DETOXIFICATION becomes important when you believe that **TOXIFICATION** is a reality. **TOXIFICATION** refers to the accumulation of toxic wastes in the cells of the body so that normal function is distorted or prevented. **TOXIFICATION** refers to the accumulation of toxic wastes that denies adequate nutrients to nourish organs and tissues. **WHEN TOXIFICATION EXISTS. . .YOU BECOME ILL!!!**

THE FOLLOWING ARE WAYS YOU ACCUMULATE TOXINS:

1. **EXTERNAL TOXINS** are various non-food substances taken into the body like the chemicals in food, water, air, and synthetics. A newspaper article written 15 years ago said we had formulated our 200,000th chemical (now over 7,000,000). *"PROGRESS" MEANS*

NEW CHEMICALS ARE BEING FORMULATED ALL THE TIME FOR THE "NEW AND IMPROVED" OBSESSION WE HAVE IN THIS COUNTRY.

The body is capable of making most normal chemical exposures inert and storing them in the body, or excreting them through the elimination systems. *THIS TAKES ENERGY "BORROWED" FROM NORMAL BODY FUNCTION, AND ALLOWS LESS NUTRIENTS AND BODY ENERGY FOR THE ACTIVITIES THAT KEEP YOU HEALTHY.*

2. **COMBINED CHEMICALS** IN THE SYSTEM MAY BE MORE DANGEROUS THAN ANY OF THEM SINGULARLY. There are second and third generations of combined chemicals that have had virtually no research done on how they affect the body.

3. **BY-PRODUCTS OF METABOLISM ACCUMULATE** WITHIN THE CELLS BECAUSE OF POOR INTRACELLULAR ENERGY AND DEHYDRATION. THIS CAUSES CONGESTION, LIKE FIVE O'CLOCK RUSH HOUR.

Your cells are activated by ATP (adenosine tri-phosphate) which is activated by glucose and oxygen. ATP activates your sodium and potassium pump that is the "electrical" energy of your cell. Potassium is high on the inside of a cell, and low on the outside. Sodium is low on the inside of a cell, and high on the outside. Minerals have a magnetic pull from high to low, so potassium is always trying to get out, and sodium is always trying to get in. The sodium-potassium pump keeps these minerals in balance in the cell by "jerking" potassium in if it goes out, and "jerking" sodium out if it goes in. This jerking action produces the electrical energy of your cells in the same way a temporary magnetic field changing direction from North pole to South pole, induces an electromagnetic field (EMF) producing electrical energy. Without electrical energy activating intracellular energy, your cells would not be able to utilize nutrients correctly. Anyone with low energy, chronic or acute health problems, overweight or underweight, has one degree or another of low intracellular energy.

4. **WASTE PRODUCTS ACCUMULATE THAT SHOULD BE ELIMINATED BY THE EXCRETORY ORGANS.** This causes a toxic overload on the system, like two lanes of traffic being directed to one lane. The whole body is interrelated, and all systems need to help each other out for best body function. *ANYTHING* you can do to protect the excretory organs is actually detoxifying the body. If one area is unhealthy, it puts a tremendous strain on the other areas.

THE EXCRETORY ORGANS ARE:

LUNGS:

Lungs depend upon proper breathing to take in oxygen, which is the first requirement of life. A deep inhalation floods your 750 million air sacs with new oxygen. Deep exhaling eliminates toxic gases filtered from the blood passing through the lungs. BREATH IS LIFE! When we forget how to breathe, we start dying. You must understand the importance of fresh air and correct breathing. Breathe from the diaphragm, *NOT THE UPPER LUNGS*, to get the full benefit of the body's assistance with air exchange. You should deep breathe at least five times, four times a day.

If you have chronic respiratory symptoms you need to check out allergies as a possible cause. Work on rebuilding the immune system and balancing the pH to improve the health of the lungs . . .DRINK YOUR WATER; AND ELIMINATE MUCUS-FORMING MILK, DAIRY PRODUCTS, BEEF, LAMB, AND PORK!

If you live in a new home, trailer, work in a new office, live or work with a smoker, or live in environmental air pollution you need to consider extra antioxidants A, C, E, zinc, and selenium. Check your health food store for antioxidant formulas. Grape seed extract or Pycnogenol are now popular antioxidants; there are antioxidant herbal formulas. More on this in the Internal Energy chapter.

You need to eat a diet that does not feed and encourage overgrowth of Candida yeast and parasites, as both organisms favor the lungs, and can be very destructive to the lung cells. TAKE A PARASITE DIE-OFF PRODUCT THREE TIMES A YEAR!

KIDNEYS:

The kidneys need eight glasses daily to do their job; 10 glasses in any inflammatory stage. **DO NOT LET YOURSELF GET THIRSTY!**

Over 4000 quarts of blood are filtered daily by the kidneys. The kidneys have three functions:

* To prevent dehydration and maintain normal water balance.
* To form urine, to throw off waste products.
* To keep the body from becoming too acid or too alkaline.

Some people absorb water differently, and because of hereditary factors will become easily OVER HYDRATED. If you are overweight and have overweight relatives, you should evaluate whether you are a **HYDRIPHERIC TYPE**. This is discussed in *THE CHEMISTRY OF MAN* by Bernard Jensen. Evaluate the following, and if you say "yes" to half or more of the list, consider the treatment recommendations:

- *Emotions are calm, easy-going, gentle, compassionate*
- *Diet preferences include soup, juicy dishes, and liquids*
- *Odors are easily detected, critical judge of food. Highly developed sense of touch, hearing, and smell.*
- *Imaginative and suffers in secret. A hydripheric type does not show emotions, fantasizes, has few friends besides close family, is subject to jealousy and may never get over love disappointments.*
- *Concerned with trivial happenings rather than major events. Disappointments cannot be forgotten or forgiven.*
- *Systems waterlogged and weakened causing poor digestion and absorption of nutrients. Illnesses are exhaustive.*
- *Metabolism is abnormal due to excessive tissue moisture; brain is sluggish.*
- *Appears healthy and robust but is actually ill and lacking vitality; resistive and recuperative powers are low.*
- *Joints and muscles are structurally weak.*
- *Reproductive system is weak; menses heavy or irregular.*

- *Susceptible to heat and light; easily chilled.*
- *Soft, delicate skin that is predisposed to skin and scalp diseases.*

TREATMENT:

- The biggest problem in obesity is too much starch in the diet. This excess starch changes the endocrine glands and also some glands in the intestines. This causes the intestines to turn almost all food into **sugar**. Herbal laxatives are suggested if you are constipated. The most consistent advice according to Edgar Cayce is pure grape juice. Two parts grape juice are mixed with one part water and taken 1/2 hour before **each** meal. The grape sugar will not cause weight gain and will satisfy the body's excess craving for sugar. As a result, less food will be taken at each meal. In addition, the intestinal cells that turn everything to sugar will eventually be healed.
- High vegetable diet **except** starchy vegetables like white potato, sweet potato, peas, corn, and beans.
- Foods high in organic sodium and chlorine help reduce cellular water. If you rotate all organic fruit, vegetables, nuts, seeds, and proteins, you will get organic sodium and chlorine in your diet. Use solar or sun evaporated seasalt.
- Total water intake including soup, cold or hot drinks, should be <u>no more</u> than six glasses per day.
- Fats should be severely limited except for Essential Fatty Acids in whole grains, cold-pressed oils, nut and seeds, or supplements like Flaxseed or Black Currant Seed oil.
- Protein foods are okay, but not red meat due to poor digestion.
- Short showers, no baths, saunas, whirlpools or swimming.
- Exercise daily, a minimum of 15 minutes of bouncing-type exercise, because Hydripheric types have lymphatic obesity (enlargement of lymph glands). Discussed in Internal Energy chapter.
- Some people may do better in a dry climate.

SKIN:

The skin is the hardest working organ of elimination struggling against:

- synthetic clothing that does not breathe. Recommend that clothing be cotton, wool, silk, or vicose rayon (some inexpensive rayons are synthetic).
- invisible layers of toxins that are not removed by daily skin brushing. Body brushing:

    - removes dead layers of skin and impurities.
    - opens and keeps the pores clean.
    - revitalizes and increases eliminative capacity of skin.
    - stimulates glands.
    - stimulates nerve endings and rejuvenates nervous system.
    - contributes to healthy muscle tone and fat distribution.
    - rejuvenates the complexion.
    - improves general health; helps prevent premature aging.
    - reduces microscopic mites in your bedding.

- lack of perspiration due to insufficient exercise.
- chlorine in city water that is very drying and can cause skin rashes.
- a coating of cremes that clog cells rather than healing from the inside out. Many commercial products contain the wrong kind of alcohols, waxes, and rancid animal products that produce drying and promote inflammatory problems. Suggest you call Arbonne cosmetics, 800-ARBONNE for your local distributor. This line is the purest cosmetic line available.
- poor nutrition, digestion, and elimination; and not enough **water**.
- free radicals created by the sun's ultraviolet radiation penetrates the skin, and damages the cells. You should wear a sunscreen even in the winter.

The top of your skin is made up of a tough material that forms a barrier against life-threatening organisms. While it is protecting you, it is disappearing right before your eyes. The entire population of cells in your skin is replaced once a month.

To conserve heat, the skin constricts blood vessels, raises body hair and the skin around the hair causing "goose bumps." To cool you, the skin dilates blood vessels and activates the sweat glands which lowers temperatures on the skin, and the blood near the surface. This cooled blood flows back into the system and cools other areas of the body. Your skin works hard for you and deserves the best cosmetic line, eight glasses of water daily, a good daily brushing, and chlorine-free bathing.

LIVER: (already discussed in the Digestion chapter).

BOWEL:

The bowel is your sewage system of your body; by abuse and neglect the bowel can become dangerously foul!!!

OF LESSER IMPORTANCE BUT STILL PART OF ELIMINATION are secretions from eyes, ears, nose, throat, and emotions of anger, joy, and sorrow.

> *ACCUMULATION OF TOXINS IN ALL THESE AREAS PRODUCE A SIMILAR RESULT: DISTORTED, DELAYED OR PREVENTED CELLULAR ACTIONS THAT ARE NECESSARY FOR THE PREVENTION OF DISEASE . . . AND FOR THE PROTECTION OF LIFE.*

[] [] [] [] [] []

YOU, THE UNIQUE INDIVIDUAL

The way a person deals with emotional or mental stress, the amount of exercise, and positive thinking, are important factors in how each person deals with the PHYSICAL STRESS of *ACCUMULATED TOXINS*. Each person's body reacts uniquely to toxic stress, so one person with toxicity may develop arthritis, another cancer.

Periodically the body tries to cleanse itself by various "acute" conditions like the common cold or flu. Stress is very important, and can put the system already toxic into rebellion. Only those with a "ripe" toxin accumulation that needs to be eliminated at that particular time will develop a cold or infection. **LEARN TO TUNE INTO BODY LANGUAGE. A COLD IS NOT BAD LUCK. IT IS YOUR BODY TELLING YOU THAT YOU ARE TOXIC, AND YOUR IMMUNE SYSTEM IS DOWN!!!**

THE MAJOR CAUSE OF TOXEMIA IS CONSTIPATION...
THE BIG C!

Even before the health of this country got so out of hand, Harvey Kellogg, M.D. of Battle Creek, Michigan (sound familiar?) performed over 20,000 operations, and found less than 10 percent of the patients had healthy colons.

THE CHOICE IS YOURS NOW! YOU CAN PAY THE HIGH COST FOR THE TREATMENT OF DISEASE, OR ASSIST YOUR BODY IN MAINTAINING HEALTH BY EATING AND DIGESTING HEALTHIER FOOD, AND INCREASING ELIMINATIONS NATURALLY.

Nature is the only one who cures. The best we can do is to help, and not hinder. We can immobilize the fracture with a cast, but it is not the cast that heals the fracture; the body heals itself. We should learn not to use modern medicine's arsenal unless it is an emergency. Once stable, go back to fundamentals so you cure the root of the problem - not just knock off one of the branches.

☐ ☐ ☐ ☐ ☐ ☐

AS MUCH AS 90 PERCENT OF ALL DISEASES START WITH PROBLEMS IN THE INTESTINE. WE SADLY KNOW MORE ABOUT TUNING OUR CARS THAN WE DO ABOUT OUR BODIES.

Africans, with their high-fiber vegetable diet and large, wet, unformed stools have little hospital huts. The constipated Americans, with their red meat, white bread, and small tubular stools, have multi-story hospitals. Most people living in modern society today are constipated with one or both of the following types:

- *One type is present when the feces that pass from the body are overly packed together.*
- *Another type is present when old, hardened feces stick to the colon walls, and do not pass out with regular movements.*

Both types are so common in our society that scarcely anybody recognizes them as being unnatural. Many people consider

ANY daily, or every other day movement (regardless of the amount) as normal; and few people have any idea how much old, hardened feces are present in their bodies.

[] [] [] [] [] []

POSSIBLE PROBLEMS FROM WASTE PRODUCT ACCUMULATION IN THE COLON:

- **ALTERNATING DIARRHEA AND CONSTIPATION** because our American diet is like glue. Mucus-forming substances adhere to the intestinal walls, and as each layer develops, the tissues become thickly covered and less functional. Diarrhea can simply be a bad condition where the intestine is so badly clogged that the solids are held back; with only a small hole open, just the liquids are getting thorough. The "virus bug" and bad food get blamed for a lot of diarrhea! abdominal pain and cramps often clear up after the laxative and enema preparations needed for X-ray exams. The doctor can find nothing wrong, and may order unnecessary drugs that will never help until the CAUSE of constipation is addressed.

- **LOW BACK PAIN** may be caused by toxic poisons retained in the bowel, irritating the nerves.

- **HEADACHES** that are not explained by dehydration, food allergies, chemical sensitivities, Candida yeast, or parasites may improve as the system is detoxified.

- **FATIGUE** from general toxic build-up.

- **REDUCED LEVELS OF THE B VITAMINS** produced in the colon.

- **INTERFERENCE WITH THE ABSORPTION OF NUTRIENTS** into the bloodstream.

- **IRRITATED NERVE ENDINGS** that can lead to spastic or inflammatory conditions.

- **TOXIC POISONS WHICH DETERIORATE THE WHOLE BODY** producing cellular malfunction.

- **BLOODSTREAM GETS THICK WITH MUCUS** (undigested protein), so the waste from cells cannot be removed properly.

- **BODY MUST CARRY AROUND EXTRA WEIGHT** that could be up to 10 pounds.

- **INTESTINAL MUSCLE ACTION (called peristalsis) BECOMES SLUGGISH**, and fecal material backs up. Since moisture is re-absorbed, a hard stool is formed and contributes to hemorrhoids.

- **EXPOSURE TO INCREASED LEVELS OF ESTROGEN** because excess circulating estrogen is not broken down by the liver, and excreted in the bile or urine. In chronic constipation, re-absorbed toxins puts such a load on the liver, it cannot properly break down excess circulating estrogen. Added to the "look-alike" chemical estrogens, this can create many health problems. Practically every man and woman on the planet is being exposed to certain environmental pollutants like PCB, dioxins, DDT (still a threat in the soil), synthetic chemicals and detergents that all "mimic" the effects of estrogen in the body. Correcting constipation is a very important step in preventing breast cancer, or one of the other estrogen-dependent cancers.

[] [] [] [] [] []

SIX REQUIREMENTS FOR HEALTHY ELIMINATION:

1. **Water** - Eight glasses of distilled or filtered water daily!!!.

2. **Fiber** - if you have enough fiber, your movement will be:

   - large amount (a comfortable feeling you've eliminated enough). Multiple "urgings" throughout the day with minimum elimination is not normal.
   - soft, wet and bulky (more like formed cow droppings, or soft tubular); if movement is packed tubular, YOU ARE CONSTIPATED!
   - low in odor (no airing out the room before another can enter)
   - passed quickly without straining (no magazine racks needed)
   - one time *BEFORE* noon, and perhaps another later in the day.

KINDS OF DIETARY FIBER (some foods contain both):

- **INSOLUBLE FIBER** does not dissolve; it provides bulk and helps in the movement of food and water through your intestine.
- **SOLUBLE FIBER** dissolves; it lowers cholesterol, detoxifies bile acids, controls appetite, slows absorption of glucose.

VALUES OF DIETARY FIBER:

- **Holds water and provides bulk** that moves food quickly through the digestive tract. Water and bulk combine to make fiber an effective cleanser, moving through your intestines like a sponge picking up wastes, toxic debris and pollutants along the way. The bulkier, softer stool means less strain and pressure on your bowels and their blood vessels.

- **Reduces toxic waste**, since food that is held up in the small intestine too long, due to lack of water and fiber, causes fermentation and putrefaction to occur. That toxic waste floods the bloodstream and produces internal toxemia and disease. *YOUR COLON IS NOT A STAINLESS STEEL HOLDING TANK! THE COLON CAN HOLD EIGHT OR MORE MEALS WORTH OF UNDIGESTED FOOD AND WASTE WHEN CONSUMING THE TYPICAL WESTERN DIET, COMPARED TO ABOUT THREE MEALS WITH AN ADEQUATE FIBER DIET AND ENOUGH WATER.*

- **Decreases re-absorption of bile salts** that are meant to be eliminated. This creates a need for the liver's cholesterol stores to make more bile acid, and that lowers blood cholesterol levels; also bile acid normalizes intestinal flora and decreases growth of unhealthy microorganisms.

- **Speeds elimination and decreases calories absorbed.** Excess fat and sugar is excreted, instead of raising triglyceride levels, or stressing the pancreas.

3. **Exercise** - gets nutrients to cells and removes toxic waste at a speed allowing the body to work at optimal performance or heal itself. This is discussed in the Internal Energy chapter.

4. **Balanced pH of the body**. Refer to the Digestion chapter.

5. **Control of Candida yeast and parasites.** It is very important to practice the "parasite" diet guidelines on a daily basis in your home, as a lifetime commitment to wellness. On social and special occasions, you can enjoy a favorite treat.

6. **Healthy stress management.** People want health to be easy, like getting rid of a headache with Tylenol. You may be disappointed in your results if you only work on the physical symptoms, and not deal with the emotional, mental, and spiritual needs. Deciding on a goal, building your future, putting value in your life, improving your self-esteem, and understanding your basic needs will help balance pH. . .and improve a lot more than elimination. Read Chapter 1 again!

[] [] [] [] [] []

RECOMMENDATIONS TO IMPROVE ELIMINATION

A BALANCED pH IS A PRIMARY GOAL. If your pH is not normal you must make that **top priority.** Read the Digestion chapter again. All recommendations will be temporarily successful if you do not follow the six requirements for healthy elimination.

The following recommendations are based on general health of the elimination system. If for any reason your medical history includes current problems in the stomach, intestines, liver or gallbladder, you should contact your medical doctor and have a complete evaluation. If all tests are normal but you still have symptoms, then you may want to consider one of the following:

- **Herbal laxative formulas** are available in health food stores, and through health magazines and mail order companies. Herbal formulas are not like "laxatives" that only force elimination. Herbal formulas help heal the body because they also support the health of interrelated systems. As your elimination becomes healthier, you will be able to reduce your intake of these supplements. *BE MORE CONCERNED ABOUT CONSTIPATION THAN DEPENDENCE ON HERBS.* Just a few examples are:

- Soloray Sp12 in most health food stores
- Nature's Way Naturalax 3 in most health food stores
- Swiss Kriss in most health food stores
- Innerclean Tabs in some health food stores
- Inside Out from Light Force
- Sea Farine (discussed below)

- **Natrum Muriaticum Cell Salts** will help to balance the fluid in the intestines if the movement is hard or loose.

- **Fenugreek** is an intestinal lubricant and is healing for sores, ulcers, and other irritations in the intestines. Two delicious drinks are:

   (1) 1/2 tsp. fenugreek, 1/2 tsp. mint, 1/2 tsp. comfrey, and 2 star anise in a cup of hot water with honey optional
   (2) "Traditional Medicinals" herbal tea makes "Smooth Moves".

- **Natural fiber products like psyllium seed** are available in health food stores to assist with colon cleansing. However, make **SURE** you drink eight glasses of **water** or they can seriously constipate you. My best high fiber recommendation is Sea Farine (address in the reference section at the back of the book). They will mail a pound to you for $29.00 plus postage.

> *Sea Farine is a sea plant found in tropical reef waters, hand-harvested by divers and sun dried, changing its natural bright gold, red and green colors to cream colored. It is higher in fiber and lower in calories than bran, contains most vitamins, is high in minerals (especially zinc), and is a natural source of mucopolysaccharides needed for healthy tissues. The dried form swells when softened with water. Soak 1/8 ounce (use a scale) in 1-1/2 cups filtered or distilled water overnight; then blend Sea Farine and water to a gel in a blender and refrigerate. After chilling, the consistency should be like thick*

jello that you can still pour. Increase or decrease Sea Farine as needed to get the correct consistency. Start with 1 teaspoon, increasing as needed up to 1/2 cup daily, for healthy elimination. The gel acts like Pepto-Bismol in your intestines, as it slides into tiny crevices and loosens years of dried fecal material. You may experience constipation as material loosens; take an herbal laxative to flush it out if you do not have a bowel movement before noon. DRINK WATER!!!!

- **A high fiber diet** means foods in their most natural form and unrefined:

    - Brown rice and whole grains instead of refined or processed.
    - Fresh fruit with skin and seeds if edible instead of drinking juice. Kiwi, berries, bananas, pears, apricots, peaches, cherries, pineapple, figs, and apples are high fiber fruits.
    - Cereals and breads containing high fiber and bran. Toast bran with sesame or sunflower seeds for casseroles or dessert toppings.
    - Nuts or seeds for snacks, or chopped in recipes or salads. Add flaxseeds and psyllium seeds to soups, stews, and casseroles.
    - Unpeeled potato, sweet potato, and vegetables. All vegetables contain fiber, especially dark green, leafy ones. Make sure you scrub non-organic potatoes well, and cut out all the "eyes". Potatoes can be sprayed with a fungicide, mold retardant and sprout inhibitor. . .it's best to buy organic. Carrots help to liquefy bile which is your body's natural laxative.
    - Precook beans; freeze for quick meals. Make bean soups and freeze for future meals. All dried and fresh beans (legumes) are high in fiber.
    - Seaweeds contain trace elements often missing in today's food and contain bulk cellulose for your high fiber diet. Check Oriental food stores, and health food stores for many different seaweeds.
    * There is no fiber in meat, fowl, fish, seafood, dairy, fats or oils.

- **Grapes** are excellent for secretions of bile to stimulate the intestines. Eat whole grapes with skin and seeds. Do not drink grape juice unless cleansing, due to mold content and high simple carbohydrates. If you do cleanse with grape juice, make sure you buy organic.

- Drink regularly throughout the day, and do not get thirsty. You should drink a glass of water 1/2 hour before each meal, and the rest should be spread out over the day for best hydration. Forgetting to drink and then drinking large amounts to catch up will only flush out minerals.

- **All fresh fruits and vegetables** are good for the intestines. Cooked fruits and vegetables cause great loss in potassium needed for intestinal movement, call peristalsis. If the liquid left after cooking vegetables is a small amount, drink it, or freeze and save for soups. . .do not discard those valuable minerals! Diets high in salt can cause low potassium levels that will interfere with good elimination. This is no time for the typical American fast food, microwave, and overcooked diet.

- **Blackstrap molasses** is a natural laxative. As a hot drink, put one teaspoon or more as desired in hot water. Blackstrap molasses is a source of iron and calcium. It is a simple sugar so use in moderation.

- **Prunes** create waste-washing action from their rich potassium. Prunes are simple carbohydrates so consume in moderation. Pour two cups of boiling water over a few prunes, cool, and consume before breakfast.

- **Garlic** has a laxative effect and is rich in potassium. GARLIC IS ONE OF YOUR BEST FOOD FRIENDS. Garlic dissolves wastes and propels them toward elimination channels; a powerful blood cleanser. One clove a day helps keep your bloodstream clean. Garlic supplements are deodorized; two garlic three times a day will detoxify sludge-filled blood. Best garlic supplements are Garlitrin 4000, or Kyolic brand.

> *Garlic has cleansing elements that have a beneficial effect on the entire system, from stimulating the appetite and secretion of gastric juices, to the promotion of peristalsis, to elimination of intestinal parasites, aiding the elimination of poisons from the body through the skin pores, is antibacterial and antiviral, and has a cleansing action on the kidneys.* **WHAT A FOOD!!!**

- **Aloe Vera juice** with its superior nutritive and cleansing qualities can help cure intestinal problems. Multiple months of Aloe use may be needed to turn around chronic colon conditions. It is important to check out different companies because the quality of Aloe varies greatly. *I ONLY RECOMMEND ALOE COMPANIES THAT STATE COLD-PRESSED, WHOLE LEAF, AND 10X CONCENTRATION.* If you cannot find this therapeutic quality Aloe, call 1-888-432-5477. Refer to cleansing Option #6 for instructions.

Aloe Vera has been well documented for the following uses:

- Natural cleanser.
- Relieves pain both surface and deep, including pain associated with joints and sore muscles.
- Bactericidal, when it is maintained in high concentration for several hours in direct contact with infectious bacteria.
- Virucidal under the same conditions.
- Fungicidal under the same conditions.
- Dilates capillaries, increasing blood supply in the area to which it is applied.
- Reduces the fever or heat of sores.
- Anti-inflammatory, having action similar to steroid.
- Stops itching.
- Nutritional, as it provides a wide range of nutrients, including mucopolysaccharides for healthy joints.
- Digests dead tissue including pus through the action of enzymes, hastening healing.
- Moisturizes the tissue.
- Safe to use for animals with similar problems.
- An FDA approved safe food. It has been taken internally by all ages from infant to elderly throughout the world since 400 years before Christ.

- **Olive oil** is an excellent natural laxative. It stimulates the liver, and gallbladder, and lubricates the intestines without blocking absorption. Consider taking one teaspoon two times a day in rice or soy milk; or use in cooking.

- **A relaxing defecation schedule**. Do not set the morning alarm so late that you have to rush. If you know you can't have an elimination until you eat breakfast, then eat when you first get up, and not just before leaving the house.

- **Tranquillity in eating and digestive routines.** Stress disrupts normalcy. Remember digestive and elimination systems are interrelated, and both are greatly affected by emotions.

- **Exercise** mechanically stimulates the intestines. A stooped or relaxed posture induces constipation by weakening the abdominal muscles. An erect posture secures proper exercise of the muscles of the trunk, and encourages correct breathing and healthy blood circulation. If your circulation becomes sluggish, there is a toxic buildup in your cells. Unless discomfort is due to an injury or infection, your INTERNAL TOXEMIA shows itself as PAIN.

[] [] [] [] [] []

THE INTERNAL HOUSECLEANING

A good house cleaning really helps after six months of surface dusting and vacuuming. Your intestines and entire body need extra attention twice a year also, to get rid of hidden build up of toxins, and waste products. If this sounds scary or unappealing, listen to all the options and I'm sure you will find one choice that is acceptable. You **DO** have choices. . .reduce the chances of getting sick and aging too fast. . . or dying too soon.

Some people cannot fast without food while they are cleansing because they are hypoglycemic or diabetic, underweight, too ill, too active, or need a certain level of energy for a demanding lifestyle or job. Cleansing is still possible with normal modified meals. If you are concerned based on your medical history, you should first check with your doctor. *ALL RECOMMENDATIONS SHOULD START OUT ON A LOW DOSE, AND WORK UP TO SUGGESTED DOSE AS TOLERATED!!* There is a safe cleanse for everyone. Products and books mentioned are available at most health food stores.

CLEANSING PROGRAMS WITH MUCUSLESS MEALS

CHOICE #1. Follow a modified mucusless diet outlined in *DR. CHRISTOPHER'S THREE DAY CLEANSE, MUCUSLESS DIET, AND HERBAL COMBINATIONS* (in the reference section in the back of this book). The mucusless diet followed for one month or a lifetime will provide a gentle cleansing. For the purpose of cleansing, a mucusless diet has some changes:

- Eliminate all commercial refined and processed foods.
- Eliminate refined sugar and commercial sodium chloride salt.
- Eliminate eggs.
- Eliminate red meat (beef, large wild animals, pork, lamb) and seafood.
- Eliminate milk and dairy products. Use soy milk as the best calcium source; or rice milk, oat milk, nut milk, or potato milk (Vegelicious). Better Butter allowed in moderation.
- Eliminate all refined flour products. Consume only 100 percent whole grain products which are mucus forming when cooked, but allowed because of their nutritional value and fiber.
* May have hormone and antibiotic-free chicken or turkey, rabbit, all fresh fruits, raw vegetables, cold-pressed oils, raw nuts, raw seeds, and natural sugars.

CHOICE #2. Take any intestinal cleanser product available in health food stores, health magazines or health catalogs, according to directions for one month. Make sure you drink eight glasses of filtered or distilled water daily, or one ounce of water for every two pounds of body weight. Follow a mucusless diet for one to two months.

CHOICE #3. Take either of the lemon juice cleanses in the liver section of the Digestion chapter. Follow the mucusless diet for one to two months.

CHOICE #4. Dandelion, red raspberry leaves, and thyme are good cleansing teas to add to any cleanse. The best "Spring Tonic" tea is Elder Flower, known for its ability to clean out the wastes that accumulate in your bloodstream. One Elderberry cleanse is available by calling Flora, Inc. 1-800-498-3610.

CHOICE #5. Cleanse with Sea Farine, gradually increasing amount from one teaspoon to 1/4 cup twice a day; take herbal laxative if cleansing constipates you. The amount of Sea Farine needed may vary greatly depending on the amount of other fiber in the diet. May be combined with Choice #6; follow the mucusless diet for one to two months.

CHOICE #6. Cleansing too quickly with 10X, cold-pressed and whole leaf Aloe Vera juice may cause flu-like symptoms. If you have symptoms, do not increase dose until you feel better. Take as outlined for a total of two bottles, twice a year.

DAY 1 - 1/2 Tsp 1X day   DAY 5 - 2 Tsp 3X day
DAY 2 - 1/2 Tsp 2X day   DAY 6,7,8 - 1 Tbsp 3X day
DAY 3 - 1/2 Tsp 3X day   DAY 9,10,11 - 1 1/2 Tbsp 3X day
DAY 4 - 1 Tsp 3X day   DAY 12,13,14 - 2 Tbsp 3X day

CHOICE #7. Any detoxification program will benefit from cleansing with Flor-Essence, either liquid or make your own tea at home (a similar product is called Essiac; both available in most health food stores). Recommend starting with 1/2 ounce once a day in the morning **on an empty stomach** for two days; if you have no adverse symptoms, increase to 1/2 ounce morning and bedtime for two days, then one ounce morning and bedtime, then two ounces morning and bedtime. **Only take one hour before or two hours after food.** Suggest reading *THE ESSIAC REPORT* by Richard Thomas.

[] [] [] [] [][]

BODY CLEANSES THAT REQUIRE FASTING

CHOICE #1. *DR. CHRISTOPHER'S THREE DAY CLEANSE, MUCUSLESS DIET, AND HERBAL COMBINATIONS* as discussed in the book.

CHOICE #2. Lemon juice cleanse for 1, 2, or 3 days depending on state of health, activity, work, and dedication as follows:

1. Before the fast take an herbal laxative if bowels have not been moving before noon daily.

2. Add juice of 6-10 fresh lemons to two quarts of distilled or filtered water sweetened with maple syrup or raw honey.
3. Drink only the two quarts of lemon water plus any distilled or filtered water you want. You may dilute the lemons more by adding extra water to use less sweetener, but drink it all each day. Drink four ounces every two hours, alternating with another quart of filtered or distilled water as tolerated.
4. If necessary, you may munch on raw carrots or celery.
5. Each day consume from 1/4 to two teaspoons of olive oil three times a day. If tolerated, increase to one tablespoon three times a day to cleanse the gallbladder and liver. *START OUT WITH A LOW AMOUNT TO TEST YOUR TOLERANCE.* Too rapid cleansing with olive oil will cause nausea.
6. After three days of cleansing, on Day 4, return food slowly to the system. Add fresh vegetables and fresh fruit first.
7. Day 5, add white chicken meat.
8. Day 6, add other mucusless foods; continue mucusless diet for one to two months.

CHOICE #3. Fasting should always be done with filtered or distilled water to rid the body of toxic wastes. Fasting one day a week on plain water or with lemon juice; or fresh fruit; or fresh apple or grape juice could add health filled years to the average American. Do not fast on liquids alone for more than three days; longer than one day, include olive oil so the gallbladder is also cleansed; follow a liquid cleanse with a mucusless diet for one to two months.

[] [] [] [] [] []

THINGS TO REMEMBER IN CLEANSING

- Discontinue all supplements during a **fasting** cleanse, but continue taking prescription drugs.

- If cleansing produces a cold, flu-like symptoms, or an increase in old symptoms, that is a sign of the **real need for cleansing**, as your body moves toxins out of the system. If you are too symptomatic, stop the cleanse. Follow a mucusless diet for one month, with eight glasses of water and exercises daily; then try cleansing again.

- If you do not have a bowel movement every day on a cleanse, take an enema, or herbal formulas as needed. *DO NOT CONTINUE TAKING CLEANSING RECOMMENDATIONS IF YOU ARE CONSTIPATED, NOT DRINKING EIGHT TO TEN GLASSES OF DISTILLED OR FILTERED WATER DAILY, AND EXERCISING TO MOVE THE LYMPHATIC SYSTEM.* If constipation or diarrhea is experienced, you will need to judge what program you are on to determine if changes must be made.

- You could feel weak on a cleanse as your body works hard internally. Use this time to rest and catch up on reading, TV, and hand work. Start it when you have several days off to evaluate reactions. It is important to do 15 minutes daily of lymphatic exercise options (Internal Energy chapter) during a cleanse, but no other strenuous choices, or exercise longer than 15 minutes each day.

- You did not become toxic in a few days, so be patient and realize it may take multiple cleanses to regain your health. You will find a favorite cleanse, and you should do it two times a year for *Spring and Fall housecleaning.*

- To help remember to drink on a liquid cleanse, set a kitchen timer.

- There may be weight loss due to the body discarding waste. These are all signs of building health. In health, weight will normalize. If weight loss would be a problem, you should pick a cleanse that allows you to eat a mucusless diet, rather than a **fasting** cleanse.

- You must first deal with an existing medical problem, and alter your cleanse to fit your needs. A person with Candida yeast overgrowth, allergies, diabetes, heart disease, or being treated for a disease must first think of those limitations before selecting a cleanse or modifications. *REMEMBER: ANY VERSION OF ANY CLEANSE, OR ANY LENGTH OF TIME IS BETTER THAN NO CLEANSE AT ALL. A MUCUSLESS DIET ALONE IS A CLEANSE.* If you have any concerns due to your past medical history, first check with your attending physician.

[] [] [] [] [] []

DETOXIFICATION IS CELLULAR ASSISTANCE FOR A LONGER LIFE!!! ONE OF THE BEST WAYS TO DETOXIFY YOUR BODY IS TO ADD OXYGEN!!!

Too many people breathe shallow breaths, and do not exercise enough to encourage deep breathing. The earth's oxygen supply is rapidly being reduced with rampant deforestation. Add to that overeating, mineral deficiency, the dangerous additive fluoride in our water, and you have a body starved for oxygen. The results of "oxygen depletion" are fatigue, depression, loss of concentration, poor judgment, irritability and a long list of chronic and acute health problems. People die in their own waste. You can put a sack over your head and be dead very quickly. THE ONLY WAY YOU ARE GOING TO LIVE A HEALTHY LIFE IS TO REMOVE THOSE WASTES FROM YOUR BODY!!!

WE LIVE OR DIE ON A CELLULAR LEVEL; the cleaner your bloodstream and your lymphatic system, the healthier your body. Every part of your body is washed, nourished, and oxygenated by your bloodstream every second of your life. Without a supply of clean, oxygenated blood, your tissues and cells will age. . .and die.

The substance that removes waste in the planet is ozone. Oxygen is a two molecule atom, and ozone is a three molecule atom. The third molecule combines with a pollutant, and oxidizes it, which converts the pollutant to another form that is not damaging. The ozone level is considered a level of pollution, but it really is the planet's ability, or lack of it, to protect itself from the build-up of pollution. High ozone levels also mean high pollution. Ozone is a very powerful oxidizer. As early as World War I it was used in the treatment of wounds. It has become an alternative to chlorination, being used in the largest ozone water purification center in the world in Los Angeles.

The same process happens in your body when ozone is applied to a virus, bacteria, fungus or plant physiology. . .it oxidizes it, and destroys it. If you had enough oxygen in your body, it would produce the ozone needed, because the electrical charges in your body actually produce ozone. Ozone acts as a beneficial scavenger, efficiently destroying diseased cells and invading organisms through the oxidation process.

An example of slow oxidation is rust, and fast oxidation is fire. In the body some types of oxidation are harmful, and produce free radicals. Your best protection against the damage of "negative" oxidation is to take antioxidants like Vitamin A, E, C, zinc, selenium, Q10, and SOD. This is discussed more in the Internal Energy chapter. *NEVER TAKE AN OXYGENATING PRODUCT WITHOUT ANTIOXIDANTS!* We know there would be no life if certain oxidation did not occur. The body uses oxidation as its first line of defense against bacteria, virus, yeast, and parasites. Without oxidation we die very quickly.

One good way to supply extra oxygen is hydrogen or magnesium peroxide ingestion. Everyone knows about hydrogen peroxide, but few people know how powerfully it can heal. Health food stores carry books that will educate you on the value of oxygen products. Many supplement companies are now producing oxygen products with enthusiastic information and testimonials. Many products are worth your consideration, but remember. . .always take them with an antioxidant formula. Hydrogen peroxide is not a cure-all, but incredible successes have been well documented in dozens of conditions. It is up to the individual to investigate all opportunities to encourage body healing in a way that "first does no harm". That is what self-responsibility in health care is all about.

[] [] [] [] [] []

Self-responsibility in health care would not be complete without knowledge of general exercise, and the **right kind of exercise for the lymphatic system.** You are getting close to the end of your beginners course in wellness, so to complete your metamorphosis. . .read on. . .

CHAPTER 5

INTERNAL ENERGY

If I told you all you needed for good health was a daily banana split, you'd probably rush to the nearest ice cream store. . .and you would *LOVE* my book! We would all like health to be easy. . .and fun. . .but, if you are like many people, you may believe that is not possible. Well, you're wrong. . .health can be easy. . .and fun!!!

Many school age children love Physical Education class. They don't realize that their happy positive attitude and deep breathing is good for their health. Too often, those playful children mature into serious, goal-oriented adults. If we lose our youthful enthusiasm for life, it can become very difficult to establish exercise habits just for enjoyment. The exercise we do establish is often associated with social or business opportunities.

At about age 40, or sooner, our bodies begin to slow down. Unfortunately, just about the time you realize you have lost a degree of health, you may be too sick, too tired, or too overextended in your lifestyle to make healthy choices. **If you are not in any acute state of poor health, you may decide to put things off until tomorrow. . .or, bad problems happen to the other guy.** When problems do happen you may be too willing to let the medical professional keep you going with a "quick fix". IF YOU DID LOSE CONTROL OF YOUR HEALTH. . .IT IS SIMPLY A MATTER OF CHOICE TO GET CONTROL BACK! Following the laws of wellness, drinking eight glasses of water and exercising daily is the place to start.

It's not important what you play. . .it's just important that you play. Play may be the most vital thing you do! FITNESS is the key word to enjoying life to the fullest, on all levels of physical, emotional, mental and spiritual. There are many books available that recommend exercise to overcome the tendency towards overweight, poor circulation, constipation, and multiple diseases. THIS CAN HARDLY BE CONSIDERED FUN!!! FITNESS SHOULD BE A LOT MORE THAN PREVENTING DISEASE. . .IT SHOULD ALSO BE FUN!!!

[] [] [] [] [] []

WHAT MAKES ONE PERSON EXERCISE, AND ANOTHER SHOW NO INTEREST?

Your decision to exercise is based on more than your physical condition. It is your state of TOTAL WELLNESS...like getting up in the morning and looking forward to the day. You may not have any physical symptoms, but you may still be unmotivated; if you have emotional or mental symptoms YOU JUST DON'T CARE TO EXERCISE! Negative emotions or negative thinking can interfere with your *enthusiasm*, even if you are free of physical symptoms. Acute problems are generally on the physical level, but most other times, symptoms are mental or emotional as well as physical. Learn how all these levels influence your life, and it will help you understand why you make certain choices.

> ***MENTAL PROBLEMS*** *are thinking problems. Thought processes can have a powerful influence on our motivations. A positive thought might be, "I think it is a great idea to go." A negative thought might be, "I don't think I'm up to going." Negative mental thinking can inhibit your ENTHUSIASM.*
>
> *There is a difference between poor mental health and poor mental attitude. You may need medical supervision for mental illness, but you can decide through WILL AND DETERMINATION to improve your ATTITUDE. Use the affirmations in Chapter 1. It will always be easier to consider fitness when you are coming from POSITIVE ENERGY.*
>
> *With dehydration, the level of energy in the brain is decreased, and many symptoms like fear, anxiety, insecurity, emotional problems and depression can become a major deterrent to healthy choices. A depressive state caused by dehydration can lead to chronic fatigue...and that can greatly affect the desire to exercise.*
>
> ***EMOTIONAL PROBLEMS*** *are feeling problems. Unfulfilled basic emotional needs lead to frustrations that can affect enthusiasm. POSITIVE EMOTIONS lead to happiness and the desire for social contact, motivation and physical activity. NEGATIVE EMOTIONS lead to unhappiness and withdrawal.*

You might cancel an intended walk after a disagreement with a friend. . .and none of the excellent books on exercise will make a difference in your decision. If you are emotionally upset, you are very likely to decide not to walk at all.

PHYSICAL PROBLEMS *in our society have become the comfort zone for excuses. Emotional and mental states are generally not necessary to mention, because giving an excuse that you have a headache is so socially acceptable. You are much more likely to say to someone you do not want to be with, "I'm too tired", rather than, "I'm upset with you." THIS EASY PHYSICAL EXCUSE IS USED ANYTIME YOU DO NOT WANT TO DEAL WITH A PROBLEM.*

[] [] [] [] [] []

HOW DO YOU DEVELOP ENTHUSIASM TO BE A PARTICIPANT IN LIFE?

1. Start every day with **POSITIVE THOUGHTS AND AFFIRMATIONS.** When you open your eyes in the morning, think about the miracle of being alive. *THIS IS YOUR DAY! WHAT ARE YOU GOING TO DO WITH IT?*

2. Everyday, **BE WILLING TO BE FLEXIBLE.** When petty irritations get you down, allow yourself the luxury of only a short negative period. Since nothing can be done in a negative state, the sooner you think more positively, the sooner you can get on with life. It is your *CHOICE* how you interpret your daily events.

3. Everyday, attempt to **DISCOVER WHY YOU DO NOT FEEL WELL,** instead of suppressing and masking chronic symptoms with drugs. There is a need for medical professionals to work together. In an acute crisis, modern medicine's approach is comforting, and can be life saving. After the crisis, we must always look for the *CAUSE* if the body was not working at optimum performance.

4. Everyday, **BE OPEN TO NATURAL TREATMENTS** that *improve* your constitution. . .*YOUR VITAL ENERGY FORCE!*

If you have a symptom, your vital force is down! It is your depressed vital force, not your symptom, that is the origin of disease. To change your level of health you must change your constitution or "VITAL FORCE", a subtle governing energy that organizes and directs physical and chemical action in the body. Efficiency of your vital force is reflected in degrees of health or illness.

Symptoms are an expression of your vital force's effort to heal. Do not suppress your body's attempt to communicate with you!!! Learn to tune into body language!!! Drugs that suppress symptoms should be avoided if possible, and only used in acute situations. Just treating symptoms is masking the fact that your vital force is down; you need to deal with that, rather than just temporarily wanting to feel better.

FACTORS THAT INDIRECTLY AFFECT VITAL FORCE:

- Therapy or medication for mental symptoms:

A natural way to treat mental and emotional symptoms is with Bach Flower Remedies. They are in the same category as other subtle methods of healing, and are available in health food stores. The Bach Flower remedy system heals by restoring harmony in awareness; they act more on the energy system rather than the physical body.

The healing energies are released from the flowers in a way that there can be no overdose, no side effects, and no incompatibility with any other treatment. To use flower remedies requires no training, but only the ability to acknowledge your thoughts and feelings. There is no true healing unless there is a change in outlook, peace of mind, and inner happiness.

IF THIS DOES NOT SOUND PROBABLE, THEN UNDERSTAND AND ACCEPT BACH FLOWER REMEDIES HEAL IN A WAY THAT "FIRST DOES NO HARM". Simplicity has to do with unity, perfection and harmony. That is the reason everybody feels attracted to the "simple things in life". The further your research advances, the greater you will realize the back-to-basics simplicity of all creation.

- **Psychotherapy, counseling, or Bach Flower Remedies** for emotional symptoms.

- **Supplements; medication for acute symptoms; food, chemical, or environmental testing and treatment; chiropractic and other alternative health care programs** that improve body function; and other forms of therapy for physical symptoms.

One way to give your vital force a boost and improve your sense of well-being is to increase physical and mental energy with negative ions. Ions are charged molecules of air. Over open land there are about equal numbers of negative and positive ions. When that balance is disturbed, there is trouble for all forms of life. Sprawling cities, automobiles, pollution, smoking, modern synthetic fibers, new building materials, chemical products, modern transportation, central heating and cooling systems in sealed office and apartment buildings, all are part of the man-made environment that has too few ions of both kinds for healthy, normal life.

Atmospheric ions can affect your health, well-being, efficiency, emotions, and mental attitude. Negative ions are called "happy ions", and positive ions are "grouchy ions". An estimated 60% of the population of North America spends about 80% of its time in cities and urban areas where the total ion count is hopelessly depleted.

So, if you live and work in our "new and improved world", are tired, fight with the family, suffer from tension, anxiety and depression, have erratic days and listless nights with below par sexual interest, you may be suffering from an overdose of positive ions. Some people are far more sensitive than others.

The most noticeable beneficial effect of using negative-ion generators is to repair the damage done by man himself to the air we breathe, and the world in which we live and work. Negative ions are unlikely to cure anyone of anything. Their most noticeable effect, however, is to give us more energy, both mental and physical, and improve our sense of well-being. Check health food stores and health magazines for sources of generators.

FACTORS THAT DIRECTLY AFFECT VITAL FORCE:

- Acupuncture:

Acupuncture creates a smooth flow of vibratory energy throughout the body by connecting with points on the pathways which relate to various organs, glands, and cells. Fine needles are inserted at certain points identified with body symptoms. By changing their distorted vibrational nature, balance is restored and the body can repair itself.

- Spiritual healing:

Faith and hope have performed miracles for many who have a strong spiritual connection. To experience that connection opens up new strengths.

- Homeopathy:

Homeopathy works on the principle of RESONANCE, like when a singer shatters glass on a special note that *matches* the energy of the glass. The source of a homeopathic remedy (like an herb) is "proven" to have certain symptoms when taken in excess. When these symptoms *match exactly* the symptoms of the person with a problem, the *two energies* when combined will increase the overall energy (called resonance). This increased energy raises your vital force and you are now stronger to overcome the symptoms. The importance in homeopathy is to match *alike symptoms* as much as possible on *all levels of physical, emotional, and mental.* The closer the match, the stronger the resonance. You will have no effect from the wrong remedy because there will be no resonance (like a singer who does not break glass).

I always carry an emergency kit of homeopathic and herbal ointments and formulas for sudden cold or flu symptoms, and injury or pain. You can start injury healing immediately if you use homeopathics and ointments with Arnica.

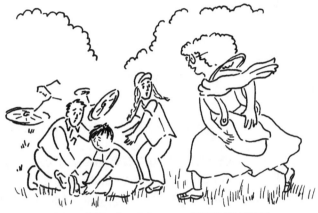

MOVE OVER! I'm an HERBALIST!

5. Everyday **THUMP YOUR THYMUS GLAND**. The word thymus is derived from the Greek work "thymos", which denotes life force. The thymus gland is strongly influenced by six major factors: stress, emotional attitudes, physical environment, social environment, food, and posture.

   Place three fingertips into the indent of your neck, at the top of your breastbone. Slide fingers down on your breastbone one inch; tap the area with your fingers for about one minute, to energize your thymus. Repeat frequently for acute symptoms.

6. Everyday be **FORGIVING OF YOURSELF AND OTHERS**! Destructive thoughts deplete your life energy...*LOVING THOUGHTS INCREASE YOUR LIFE ENERGY!*

7. Everyday stand up straight...**THINK AND WALK WITH CONFIDENCE!** This is a positive energy factor. Good posture facilitates the energy flow through the body.

8. Everyday **REACH OUT TO SOMEONE**. Be willing to touch, show affection to someone, be caring and compassionate. Outstretched arms (as in reaching out) use both right and left brain for balance. Say *"I love you"* often to someone special.

9. Everyday put the kind of **MUSIC IN YOUR LIFE** that you enjoy. The enjoyment music gives you encourages a sense of peace and calm, and that makes you want to accomplish something.

10. Everyday create **POSITIVE ENERGY**, because it can influence you and those around you. *ENERGY IS CONTAGIOUS!* A weak person can make you weak, and an energetic person in the room can energize you, *raising your life energy.*

11. Everyday dress in a way that will **TURN YOURSELF ON!**

12. AND. . .**EVERYDAY SMILE!** *LIFE IS WONDERFUL IF YOU "THINK" IT IS!!!* Your day may have a harsh challenge in it, but that should be an opportunity for learning, and not for holding on to negative thoughts..

[] [] [] [] [] []

I HAVE A GOOD ATTITUDE, I'M READY. . .WHERE DO I START?

Start by looking at exercise as a pleasant way to add relaxation to life's stressors, and add pleasure to your day. The success of your exercise program does not depend on the exercise book you are reading. . . but, on your *FRAME OF MIND!* Make a commitment to your future. Exercise is a private satisfaction; exercise is something you do for **you**. If you do not give *"YOU"* a part of each day, look at what value you place on yourself. Are you coming from "I can't be happy, and life is hard"? Ballroom dancing is an exercise treat I give to myself. You should exercise for health's sake. . .but also for pleasure. The two are self-supporting; the healthier you are, the more you'll like to exercise, and the more you like to exercise, the healthier you'll be.

[] [] [] [] [] []

FITNESS MYTHS:

Misconceptions keep people from becoming fit and healthy, such as:

- No pain, no gain.
- A person has to sweat to get in shape.
- Big muscles are important.
- Lots of protein makes a person strong.
- You must spend at least 10 hours a week in a fitness program to stay in shape.

KEY POINTS IN ACHIEVING FITNESS AND PROLONGING LIFE EXPECTANCY:

- **LOWERING THE AT-REST HEART RATE:** That rate is determined by your level of activity maintained during the last four weeks. Simply by monitoring the heart beat, the level of effort and fitness can be determined at any point in time. The mortality rate for adults with resting pulse rates over 92 is four times greater than for those with pulse rates less than 67. You should take your resting pulse when you first wake up **before you move**. Find your pulse on your wrist (the thumb side of your hand); or on your neck (straight down from your cheek bone).

- **REGAIN FITNESS IN ONE MONTH**: 80% of an individual's fitness can be gained or lost in a 28 day period. A person who hasn't exercised in years, can regain fitness in one month by following some simple guidelines.

FIVE DAILY REQUIREMENTS FOR MAINTAINING FITNESS according to Lawrence Morehouse, director of the Human Performance Laboratory at U.C.L.A.:

1. Limbering includes two or three minutes of simple stretching, twisting, bending and turning.
2. Standing for a total of two hours during the day.
3. Lifting something heavy for at least three minutes.
4. Walking briskly for at least three minutes.
5. Any activity that will burn at least 300 calories a day. The list is

long, but generally plan on something that keeps you moving at least 45 minutes.

IN ADDITION, SPREAD OUT THE FOLLOWING THREE TIMES DURING THE WEEK:

- One or two minutes of warm up, then five minutes of exercise that works the upper body, abdominal and legs.
- Five minutes of aerobic exercise that gets the pulse into the target range. This formula is for people who can safely increase their heart rate (check with your doctor if you are not sure):

Subtract your age in years from 220, and take 80 percent of that number to get your maximum heart rate. Healthier circulation will carry vital nutrients to all of your body structures, and eliminate toxic wastes. Do not exercise to exhaustion. In fatigue, you lose muscle strength three times faster than you build it. Regular exercise is safer; it builds stamina that protects you from sudden exertion that can be damaging or even fatal.

[] [] [] [] [] []

It can be a challenge to move if your back, neck, joints, and muscles hurt; some **ROOT CAUSES** are:

*- In the spinal column, water acts as a lubricant for contact surfaces, and supports 75 percent of the weight of the upper body. Once arthritis in any joint is established, it can be a lifetime sentence, unless the **ROOT CAUSE** is understood. Joint pain should be considered as **local thirst**. In a well-hydrated cartilage surface of joints, friction damage is minimal.*

*- Another **ROOT CAUSE** of arthritis is from inorganic minerals. Your body cannot assimilate inorganic calcium and potassium minerals in well, spring, and city water. Most of these minerals pass out of the body, but some slough off into the joints and build up deposits; well, spring, mineral, or city water is not recommended. If you are not drinking*

distilled or reverse osmosis water, your filter choice is only a good one if it eliminates fluoride and microscopic parasites.

- *Emotions can be a **ROOT CAUSE** of many physical symptoms. Holding resentments can be a factor in arthritis; stress can be a factor in muscle pain and general fatigue. Read Chapter 1 again!*

- *An unhealthy diet must be a main consideration for **ROOT CAUSES** in any state of ill health. If you are not faithful to a healthy diet, you may not progress at a speed that makes you want to consider exercise options. Really work at improving your absorption of food. There is a real difference between eating and getting the nutrition into the cells. KNOW WHAT YOUR pH IS EVERY MONTH THE REST OF YOUR LIFE!*

IF YOU CAN BREATHE, YOU CAN EXERCISE!

Physical restrictions may limit your physical choices, but *mental and emotional attitudes may be far more inhibiting.* Start with DEEP BREATHING and POSITIVE AFFIRMATIONS:

To deep breathe, push your stomach muscles out; take in all the air you can, let it out slowly until you cannot let any more air out, and your stomach muscles are pulled in. This is a full cleansing breath. BREATH IS LIFE! We learn to breathe at birth; when we forget how to breathe correctly, we start to die. Abnormal cells multiply in the absence of oxygen.

[] [] [] [] [] []

WHY DO SO MANY PEOPLE STOP EXERCISING AFTER THAT FIRST BURST OF ENTHUSIASM?

1. Some people exercise out of fear of illness. They do not exercise because they want to relax and treat themselves to some pleasure. Because *fear* is negative, it is likely they will have other negative attitudes, and find excuses not to continue.

2. Some stop because they feel good, and would rather do something else. *They often take health for granted!!!*
3. Some stop because the exercise was recommended treatment for a medical problem which has been resolved.
4. Some people are pressured by others to join them, but low self-esteem and subconscious negative thoughts soon win over.
5. Some like the choice of exercise to be more social; home equipment ceases to be fun in the garage.
6. Some feel the choice is too strenuous for their endurance level.
7. Some are unwilling to return to an exercise that resulted in an injury.
8. Some feel the choice may be too time consuming for their lifestyle.
9. Some feel the choice may be too stressful, or fearful. . .like skiing.
10. Some feel the choice may be too expensive to continue at this time.
11. Some feel the choice may be too inconvenient because they've moved.
12. Some feel the choice was not as much fun as they thought it would be. Be careful with this one. Are you coming from, "I can't be happy" and "life is hard?"

BE WILLING TO STRETCH OUT OF YOUR COMFORT ZONE TO TRY NEW ACTIVITIES. TAKE A RISK. . .BE ADVENTUROUS! ESTABLISH A PROGRAM TO FIT YOUR LIFESTYLE, AND THEN STICK TO IT UNTIL IT BECOMES HABIT!

[] [] [] [] [] []

EXERCISE OPTIONS HAVE IMPORTANT POINTS TO CONSIDER:

THE FOLLOWING EXERCISE OPTIONS ARE GOOD FOR THE LYMPHATIC SYSTEM:

- **JOGGING**: If you are not a "conditioned jogger" it may not be the best recommendation to start. If you are not in good physical health, jogging can be very stressful to the hips, knees, and ankles on paved roads and sidewalks. Jog on an athletic track or sawdust trail, wearing the best running shoes. Jog with a friend or dog for safety.

- **STATIONARY JOGGING OR AEROBICS:** Either purchase some exercise tapes, follow television exercise shows, or join a health club.

- **TRAMPOLINE**: This is a safer form of jogging; easier on your joints, and more acceptable when time or weather is a problem. Recommend 15 minutes once or twice a day; becomes more social while watching television. If you are unable to jump due to physical limitations, you can still get benefit from a trampoline. Sit with your feet on the trampoline, and let someone else do the jumping. Small trampolines are very inexpensive; I believe **everyone** should own one!

- **HIKING**: Getting back to nature is the best way to enjoy all the sensory groups. . .visual, auditory (hearing), kinesthetic (feeling), gustatory (taste with lunch or snack), and olfactory (smell). This produces the best relaxation. Joining organizations that enjoy the outdoors adds both friends and fun, such as Sierra Club, Audubon Society, or a photography club. THINK AHEAD. . .a little thought about food, water, clothing, shoes, bug protection, and emergency items are critical to the success of your adventures.

- **WALKING**: Shoes are most important; don't forget food, water, and clothing on longer walks. Walking is easier on the joints than jogging. Slow walking may be necessary at first, but fast walking is better for your lymphatic system. One way to indoor "walk" is with a treadmill.

- **ACTIVE BALL SPORTS**: If your bones, nerves, and muscles are not healthy, you may be prone to accidents in contact sports. If you have accidents due to constant aggression, it may be an example of your frustration in life.

- **DANCING**: You do not have to go to a night club to dance; turn the music on at home; put a little wiggle in your body. *LOOSEN UP . . .IT WILL HAVE A WONDERFUL EFFECT ON YOUR SELF IMAGE.* Smoke-free ballroom dancing is growing in popularity, and is my personal choice because it provides lymphatic exercise, pleasurable time with friends, is safe and friendly for singles and great for couples. ANYTHING THAT PUTS PLEASURE IN YOUR LIFE PROMOTES HEALTH BECAUSE YOU GET CIRCULATORY IMPROVEMENT FROM RELEASE OF TENSION.

- **THE CHI MACHINE AEROBIC EXERCISER FROM SUN HARMONY** improves your health and sense of well-being, by increasing oxygen levels. Because you are lying down to use this machine, people who are unable to do other exercise options can make a dramatic difference in their health, with "passive aerobic" exercise. The gentle jerking action tones the whole body. To order, refer to the reference section at the back of the book.

THE FOLLOWING EXERCISE OPTIONS ARE GOOD FOR CIRCULATION AND MUSCLE TONE:

- **BIKING**: Biking is fun; it boosts your circulatory system and reduces stress. *Always wear a helmet when biking*, because you have no control if you are hit by a car, or take a tumble from any number of other reasons. Today we jump in the car to go a block. Choose to walk or bike short distances. Best bike seat is the Biko Saddle available from 800-582-8088.

- **STATIONARY BICYCLE AND OTHER INDOOR EQUIPMENT**: Many people lose interest after the "new toy" period is over, especially if equipment is stored in an isolated area of the home. Place equipment near a television, or join a health club.

- **SWIMMING**: This is particularly helpful if you have an injury or physical limitations, because it is less physically stressful to move under water. You can stimulate your whole body by applying pressure from the water jets in a jacuzzi to your hands and feet, since all the meridians in your body terminate there. Do not stay in a hot jacuzzi more than 15 minutes; and only under the guidance of your doctor if you have high blood pressure.

- **YOGA, TAI-CHI OR OTHER STRETCHING CHOICES** do not increase heart rate; they should be used in addition to active exercise choices. They are helpful to limber up the body, release tension, improve body alignment, and flow of energy.

WE ARE ALL INDIVIDUALS. SOME ARE OLD AT 40, AND SOME ARE YOUNG AT 60. A LOT DEPENDS ON YOUR LIFETIME HABITS OF LIVING. IN PLANNING YOUR EXERCISE PROGRAM, CONSIDER YOUR LIFESTYLE, BUT

EVERYONE SHOULD HAVE AT LEAST A FEW MINUTES OF STRETCHING EXERCISES MORNING AND/OR EVENING. Do your routine the same time each day, as discipline is the key to your fitness program.

The prime essential in promoting any exercise program is good POSTURE. Poor posture can mean poor digestion, poor elimination, poor circulation, and set you up for fatigue that will sabotage your enjoyment of life. Be conscious of how you stand and sit, or work at a desk. To encourage good posture, stand with your back against the wall so your calves, buttocks, shoulders and back of head all touch the wall together. Raise both arms high overhead touching the wall . . .lower arms, relax, and repeat five times.

- **SKIING**: The key word to remember is CLASSES. To prevent injuries, make sure you have some understanding of your general state of health, and have enough instruction to develop self-confidence. I did it wrong; injuries included a fractured rib, and the same year a broken hip. If downhill or cross-country is too frightening for you, but you would love to get out in the snow, try snowshoes. If you can walk, you can snowshoe. The outdoor experience is worth it!!!

- **TIME TO EXERCISE:** If you exercise in the morning you will get almost 2/3 energy from stored fat and 1/3 from carbohydrates; in the afternoon, you will burn more carbohydrates. Burning fat is better for weight loss, so if overweight, exercise in the morning; exercise in the afternoon if you are more concerned about general health than weight loss.

IN SUMMARY, HOW DO YOU DEFINE EXERCISE?

Exercise is an activity that *enriches* the life of a person who has mental, emotional, and physical energy enough to be enthusiastic about life. The decision to exercise is based on the decision to *enjoy life to the fullest*. The desire to *begin* exercise implies a degree of health in **POSITIVE THINKING, NUTRITION, DIGESTION, AND ELIMINATION**. The decision to *continue* exercise is a definite degree of health in POSITIVE THINKING, NUTRITION, DIGESTION, AND ELIMINATION.

◻ ◻ ◻ ◻ ◻ ◻

STUDIES INDICATE THAT EXERCISE IS A DEFINITE FACTOR IN BLOOD VESSEL DISEASE

We have become oversensitive to the word "cholesterol". Your body needs cholesterol for vital body functions. The fact is, the less cholesterol you take in with your foods, the more the body makes; and the more cholesterol you take in with your food, the less your body produces (either way it will get what it needs).

Cholesterol production is a part of the cell survival system. Cholesterol makes the cell wall impervious to the passage of water, protecting cells against dehydration. Excess cholesterol production can mean cellular dehydration. After a period of improving cellular hydration ON A REGULAR BASIS, increased cholesterol production will be less required, and in time will decrease.

The restriction of cholesterol containing foods has very little to do with your cholesterol level alone. People and doctors love tests! It is easy to measure blood cholesterol, and if elevated, is often blamed for atherosclerosis, **when other causes are ignored.**

- *If total cholesterol is 160, ideal LDL is 100 or below.*
- *If total cholesterol is 200-240, LDL acceptable if 130 - 160.*
- *If total cholesterol is 240-300, high risk LDL is 160-200.*
- *If total cholesterol is above 300, there is an extreme high risk if LDL if above 200.*

It is recommended that your cholesterol and HDL ratio be UNDER five. Ex: HDL is 30, total cholesterol is 240, ratio is eight which to too high. If HDL is 80 and cholesterol 240, you have a low risk of three.

THE ARTERIES' HEROES AND VILLAINS STORY:

- *Cholesterol is manufactured in the body, mainly by the liver; it also goes to the liver from animal food you eat.*

- *In the liver cholesterol is loaded, along with triglycerides (a combination of fatty acids), into very-low density lipoproteins (VLDLs), which carry it through the bloodstream.*

- *After releasing their triglycerides into the body's tissues, VLDLs are transformed into different carriers, called low density lipoproteins (LDLs), which deliver cholesterol to the cells.*

- *Excess LDLs, rejected by the cells, help trigger the formation of plaque, which can build up in artery walls and block free blood flow.*

- *The heroes, high-density lipoproteins (HDLs) work against this process by removing excess cholesterol from blood and cells.*

- *HDL may also be able to collect cholesterol from the plaque, reversing the process that leads to heart attacks.*

- *Once filled with excess cholesterol, the HDLs may deliver some of their cargo back to VLDL carriers which then become LDL's as before.*

- *The liver removes LDLs from the bloodstream and converts cholesterol into bile acid, which is then eliminated. If not eliminated because of constipation, cholesterol can recirculate and increase cholesterol levels.*

◻ ◻ ◻ ◻ ◻ ◻

EIGHT COMMON SENSE HEALTH CHOICES FOR CIRCULATION:

MODERATION WILL ALWAYS BE THE BEST CHOICE IN THE SEARCH FOR HEALTH.

1. **BUTTER IS BETTER, AND BETTER BUTTER IS BETTER YET** (see Nutrition chapter). Butter contains important natural nutrients, and again, the word is MODERATION! Cholesterol food eaten in *moderation* is not going to be the *main* villain in atherosclerosis.

2. **AN EGG IS A FOOD CAPABLE OF PRODUCING LIFE!** According to Dr. K. Donsbach, "Eggs will not affect your cholesterol or blood vessel disease state except to lower your cholesterol and make your body more disease resistant." Remember MODERATION! Eggs contain enough natural lecithin to handle the amount of cholesterol in the egg.

3. **CHEMICAL POISONS CAN CAUSE ARTERIAL IRRITATION.** All the research on how chemicals affect our bodies may never be complete. Do not purchase foods with added chemicals, to help reduce the overall load from the chemicals you cannot eliminate in the environment. Our society's obsession with new homes, new cars, synthetic materials, and "new and improved" chemical everything puts a huge stress on the body's ability to protect itself. The protection antioxidants are more important than ever:

    - *Vitamin A captures free radicals which are unstable particles bent on damaging your cells. You need Vitamin A because of our upset balance of nature. You should not take more than 10,000 I.U. of Vitamin A daily, because excess can be damaging to the liver. Extra Vitamin A should be in the form of Beta-carotene, that can be stored in the skin, and changed into Vitamin A in the liver when needed.*

    - *Vitamin E is the supreme oxygen-efficiency nutrient. It is THE supplement to take if you want to reduce the speed of the aging process and protect life; use a dry rather than an oil product for better absorption.*

    - *Vitamin C is the key nutrient used by your body to detoxify harmful substances, and help protect your liver. During stress, greater than normal amounts are lost in the urine. Because it is also vital to intracellular energy and production of bile acid that protects the health of the gallbladder and normal intestinal flora, Vitamin C is the one supplement you should always take every day. Vitamin C's co-factors (bioflavonoids) inhibit the destruction of Vitamin C by oxidation. Buffered Ester-C with Bioflavonoids is the recommended C to use. Vitamin C, calcium, and pH balance are all interrelated.*

- ***Zinc*** *deficiency greatly affects the immune system. Zinc is a powerful antioxidant, and has many functions in digestion, enzyme production, and cellular activity.*

- ***Selenium*** *is deficient in most of our soil. It is imperative in controlling chemical sensitivities. Brown rice has 15 times as much selenium as white rice. THIS IS NO TIME FOR PROCESSED FOOD!!!*

4. **DO NOT DRINK HOMOGENIZED MILK!** The process produces an enzyme called Xanthine Oxidase that irritates the lining of the circulatory system, and is highly suspected as one beginning cause of atherosclerosis. Use goat's milk, raw milk, or small amount of dairy products or fat free milk in cooking (heat destroys Xanthine Oxidase).

5. **THE BEST DIET IS ONE OF MODERATION AND COMMON SENSE.** Avoid commercially processed foods, refined flour and refined sugar in products. Steer clear of recommendations for "low this" and "high that" (which varies from book to book anyway).

6. **AVOID CONSTIPATION!** It increases the reabsorption of bile salts that were meant to be eliminated. This lessens the need for the liver's cholesterol stores to make more bile acid, and that can raise blood cholesterol levels.

7. **DRINK EIGHT GLASSES OF WATER DAILY** *TO PREVENT INTRACELLULAR DEHYDRATION THAT ENCOURAGES THE BODY TO PRODUCE MORE CHOLESTEROL TO KEEP FLUID IN THE CELLS.*

8. **EXERCISE IS CERTAINLY NOT LAST WHEN IT COMES TO IMPORTANCE.** The benefits of a regular fitness program fall easily into three categories:

weight control - feeling of well-being - longevity

[] [] [] [] [] []

WHEN YOU EXERCISE YOU HAD BETTER KNOW HOW TO ABSORB CALCIUM

You may learn about CALCIUM the hard way after you break a bone. Once you question your level of calcium, you should do a test to determine your needs. This much is not unusual for people to consider, and they obediently take the calcium supplement. . .assuming that it is being absorbed. THIS IS AN ASSUMPTION YOU CANNOT AFFORD TO MAKE, BECAUSE CALCIUM IS THE MOST DIFFICULT OF ALL THE MINERALS TO ASSIMILATE!

Calcium is in every cell of the body. About 99 percent of body calcium is contained in bones and teeth. The kidneys produce a compound, and along with a hormone from the parathyroid regulate the release and absorption of one percent that circulates in body fluids. Calcium moves in and out of the bones with about 600-700 milligrams being exchanged each day.

From birth to about age 35 we build bone; after that we gradually lose more than is being replaced, about three to eight percent each decade. Sun exposure, good nutrition, and exercise can prevent or slow this process. *PREVENTING AND REVERSING OSTEOPOROSIS* by Alan Gaby, M.D. is an excellent book about calcium.

ROLES OF CALCIUM:

- Essential for healthy teeth.
- Helps to maintain the acid/alkaline balance of the body.
- Helps the blood to clot.
- Transports impulses along the nerves.
- Necessary for good muscle contraction.
- Important in brain functioning.

- Regulates the rhythm of the heartbeat.
- Initiation in some hormone secretions.
- Activation of enzyme reactions.

SOME SYMPTOMS OF LOW CALCIUM ARE:

- Inability to deal with stress. Calcium taken at bedtime can be a tranquilizer.
- Teeth grinding at night.
- Abnormal growth or rickets in children.
- Osteoporosis in adults.
- Convulsions.
- Cramps anywhere; muscle spasms or twitching.
- Heartbeat irregularities.
- Allergies.
- Bleeding tendencies.

[] [] [] [] [] []

UNDERSTANDING CALCIUM ABSORPTION:

1. **Exercise** is an *ESSENTIAL* part of calcium absorption. Rapid loss of calcium when not active contributes to exhaustion in bedridden people. Space program tests showed calcium loss in weightlessness regardless of the intake of calcium.
2. **Excessive physical, emotional, or mental stress** causes excretion of calcium to be greater, regardless of the amount of intake.
3. **Hydrochloric acid** is *NECESSARY* in your stomach for proper calcium absorption. On the other hand, calcium cannot be absorbed in a too acid system, **so pH balance is critical.**
4. **Normal levels of estrogen or testosterone** are necessary to absorb calcium. Aging encourages calcium deficiency because of generally low hormone levels.

Ask your doctor to order estrogen and progesterone levels. To protect against osteoporosis you need progesterone to build bone. Pregnenolone is a natural supplement that is a nutrient precursor to progesterone. You can also buy natural wild yam progesterone products that do not have side effects like those you could get from drug hormone replacements.

5. **Drugs** have varying effects on calcium absorption. Some (like antibiotics) increase the body's need for calcium, and some (like steroids) decrease absorption. Antibiotics destroy beneficial intestinal bacteria needed for calcium absorption. Following antibiotics, always re-establish healthy intestinal flora with Flora Balance, and acidophilus from health food stores.
6. **Phytic acid and oxalates** in certain foods such as grains, all legumes, rhubarb, potatoes, cauliflower, broccoli, spinach and asparagus hinder calcium absorption unless cooked, steamed or sprouted.
7. **Vitamin F (essential fatty acids)** is needed for calcium absorption. Use cold-pressed oils, whole grains, and unprocessed nuts and seeds; or take Flaxseed, Black-Currant, or Hemp oil as a supplement.
8. **Vitamin D** has a potent effect on intestinal absorption of calcium. Too many dairy products fortified with Vitamin D, and high intake of eggs and fish can cause too much calcium absorption. THERE'S THAT WORD MODERATION AGAIN! Ultra-violet light in sunlight on the skin changes a form of cholesterol to Vitamin D. You need about 30 minutes per day of sunlight for vitamin D synthesis. But, you can soak up Vitamin D all day and still be deficient if you aren't getting enough Vitamin A and Vitamin C.
9. **Phosphorus** is needed to absorb calcium, but too much phosphorus will cause calcium loss, as it takes calcium with it when excess amounts leave the body as calcium phosphate. We have a high phosphorus diet in this country with red meat, cereal, dairy, and carbonated drinks.
10. **Sodium fluoride** used by drug companies and the dental profession is a calcium antagonist. Calcium fluoride is safer, and you can buy calcium fluoride cell salts in health food stores.
11. **Abnormal fluid consumption, use of prescription or herbal diuretics** can flush minerals out through your kidneys. Drink fluids regularly throughout the day, rather than large amounts at one time.
12. **Diarrhea** can cause loss of nutrients. Evaluate food allergies, poor digestion of milk sugar, alternating constipation and diarrhea.
13. **Inherited weaknesses** are becoming more prominent each generation. Seemingly healthy children are born with toxic conditions, nutritional deficiencies, and allergies.
14. **White sugar** depletes calcium because it drives out calcium and shifts body chemistry in ways that can cause many problems.
15. **Thyroid disorders** can cause calcium loss. Check your thyroid function at home with this method ONCE A MONTH:

- *Place a thermometer next to your bed at night.*
- *Immediately upon awakening, without getting up, place thermometer snugly in your armpit and hold tightly for 10 minutes. If using digital type, remove when it beeps. Record reading, and repeat procedure for two more days.*
- *Women with menstrual cycles start on day two of the flow.*
- *Normal average readings are not below 97.6. A lower average indicates a need for thyroid evaluation.*

TO STRENGTHEN A SLUGGISH THYROID WITH NATURAL METHODS:

- *Take kelp, three-five tablets three times a day; use seaweeds in soups and stews. Kelp supplies B12 for the vegetarian; absorbs elements from the sea that almost completely mirror healthy human blood in amino acids, minerals and trace elements.*
- *Eat fish at least three times a week.*
- *Take 400-800 I.U. of dry Vitamin E daily to stimulate the pituitary gland which stimulates the thyroid.*
- *Take Spirulina blender drinks at least one time a day.*
- *Add Bee Pollen, Spirulina capsules, or Blue-Green Algae for extra nutritional support.*
- *Use cold-pressed oils high in essential fatty acids that produce prostaglandins, needed for hormone and enzyme production.*
- *Avoid caffeine and smoking because they encourage the intake of sweets that overstress the thyroid.*
- *Consume low simple carbohydrates: no refined sugar, fruit juice (unless diluted in half), dried fruit (unless in very small amounts), or refined grains. Use natural sugars in small amounts; fresh fruit once or twice a day only. Simple sugars in excess can stress the thyroid and cause people to gain weight in their abdomen, hips, and thighs (read Dr. Abravanel's book listed in the reference section). Increase complex carbohydrates such as whole grains, potatoes, starchy vegetables and legumes.*

15. **Magnesium** is calcium's co-pilot. Most anti-aging daily supplement programs will recommend both magnesium with potassium

supplements. Magnesium makes urine more solvent to hold crystals in solution for people who are prone to calcium oxalate kidney stones. Magnesium and phosphorus are minerals necessary to keep bones hard. It is doubtful you are getting enough magnesium unless you eat plenty of raw and unprocessed foods, because magnesium is extremely sensitive to heat.

16. **Commercial frozen vegetables** may contain EDTA, and this agent partially removes zinc, manganese, and calcium.
17. **Too high fiber diet** can cause anywhere from 100-400 milligrams of calcium to be lost per day. *MODERATION IN EVERYTHING!!!*
18. **A high protein diet** contributes to low calcium levels, because it causes the body to need calcium to neutralize acid conditions produced by excess protein.
19. **Vitamin K** produces a protein that attracts calcium into bone tissues. Vitamin K is poorly produced in an unhealthy intestine that has Candida yeast or parasite overgrowth, low healthy bacteria, and cellular dehydration.
20. **Boron**, a mineral long considered not essential to nutrition, is now indicated as reducing calcium loss. Some calcium supplements do contain boron, but you can get ample boron by eating pears, apples, grapes, leafy vegetables, nuts and legumes.

[] [] [] [] [] []

SOURCES OF CALCIUM:

The recommended daily allowance of calcium is set at 800-1000 milligrams; 1200-1500 milligrams per day for post-menopausal women; 400-800 milligrams per day for children. Stress and exercise levels have a lot to do with how much calcium you need, and how well it is absorbed.

The dairy association has persuaded us that milk is the best source of calcium, but it is only *one* source. Many foods with fewer digestive, mucus, allergic symptoms, and lower in phosphorus are also **excellent** sources of calcium.

> *Another problem with dairy products is strontium 90. It is a radioactive substance placed into the clouds by nuclear activity in some areas, absorbed by the grass from rain, eaten by the cows, and accepted by their mammary glands;*

then we drink the milk. The strontium 90 is accepted in the bones like calcium, and may contribute to the cause of some bone cancers. Bone meal from animals can also have strontium 90, so it is not a recommended source of calcium. ***USE DAIRY PRODUCTS AS ONLY ONE SOURCE OF CALCIUM, NOT THE MAIN SOURCE.***

Dolomite is ground rock, and not recommended with the better absorbed chelated minerals available. Tums is not a good source of calcium; two tablets are very low in biologically available calcium, and contains mineral oil and talc. It is strictly a commercial gimmick, and can mask a much more serious pH imbalance problem.

Four main types of calcium: calcium lactate is the same type found in milk (easy to digest unless you have trouble digesting milk), and best if the pH is too alkaline. Calcium gluconate (a salt from gluconic acid prepared by the oxidation of glucose) is easy to digest, but like calcium lactate, takes a large quantity to get enough daily. Calcium carbonate (a salt of carbonic acid formed in solution by carbon dioxide in water) requires stomach acid for proper breakdown, so **make sure the product has hydrochloric acid in it, or your saliva pH is not above 6.4.** Calcium citrate is bound to lemon fruit acids, and easier for the body to absorb and utilize; may be the best form of calcium supplement.

If you ROTATE all healthy foods, you are likely to consume many sources of calcium: Seeds (especially sesame), broccoli, cabbage, cauliflower, radish, blackstrap molasses, maple syrup, sardines, salmon, tuna, nuts (especially almond), soybeans, peanuts, green leaf and stalk vegetables, egg yolk, carob, shellfish and fish, asparagus, buckwheat, whole grains, tomato, potato, carrots, and figs. Eating sea vegetables four times a week will provide plenty of calcium if you do not eat dairy products. There are many varieties of seaweeds in health food stores that greatly improve the nutrition of many recipes. IN OTHER WORDS, EAT A WIDE VARIETY OF WHOLE GRAINS AND FRESH UNPROCESSED FOODS, AND YOU WILL GET YOUR CALCIUM, PLUS A WHOLE LOT MORE!!!

Two teaspoons of Tahini (sesame seed), **OR** *1/4 cup almonds can be mixed in one cup water in a blender to make a SUPERIOR calcium replacement for cow's milk.*

YOUR LYMPHATIC SYSTEM:

You cannot talk about exercise, calcium, circulation and body wellness without understanding there is more circulating in your body than just blood. The lymphatic system is less understood, yet there is twice as much lymph in the body as there is blood, and twice as many lymphatic vessels as there are blood vessels; the lymph system protects your health.

Did you ever pop a blister and notice the clear liquid inside? This is lymph, a yellowish fluid that is "squeezed" throughout the body in its own private circulation system. The lymph system is a vast system like the blood vessels, with one big difference. . .it has no heart to keep it moving. The lymph vessels are squeezed, and lymph pushed along and filtered through lymph nodes by deep breathing and specific exercises.

> *The best activity for the lymphatic system is any BOUNCING action previously discussed, or stroking of any discomfort area towards the chest. It is alright to choose an exercise two to three days a week for circulatory health, or exercise that strengthens muscle tone; that should be in addition to exercise for 15 minutes **DAILY** to move the lymph.*

As blood circulates and exchanges nutrients and hormones for waste products, it leaks fluids. These fluids must return to the blood, but first they are filtered through lymph nodes. *ANYTIME THE LYMPH BACKS UP YOU CAN EXPERIENCE PHYSICAL SYMPTOMS!!!* A clogged lymph system can mean upper respiratory infections, sinus or ear infections, throat problems, colds, tonsillitis as well as bronchitis and pneumonia, low back ache, pain anywhere, and tissue swelling. We need to keep the lymph system moving, and one way is through **THE RIGHT CHOICE OF EXERCISE.**

OTHER WAYS TO CARE FOR YOUR LYMPHATIC SYSTEM:

- **Distilled or filtered water** in the amount of eight glasses daily, or one ounce of water for each two pounds of body weight.

- **Reduce dietary fats** that can clog systems anywhere in the body, but you do need essential fatty acids.

- **Blood cleansing formulas** help clear out both toxic blood and toxic lymph conditions. Herbs like echinacea, goldenseal, capsicum, licorice root, hawthorn berries, ginger, and fenugreek tea all help strengthen and clear this extensive network. Aloe Vera that is cold-pressed, whole leaf and 10 times concentrate is an excellent blood and lymph cleanser (refer to reference list).

- **Liquid chlorophyll, green drinks with Spirulina, Blue-Green Algae, wheat or barley grass** are good lymph system cleansers.

- **Eat fresh fruits and lots of vegetables.**

- **Stimulate lymphatic drainage** in the following ways:

    1. Located at the bottom part of the breast bone is a reflex point. Vigorously rub that area for two minutes to help lymphatic drainage. This is the collection area for lymph drainage coming from the head down, or up from the feet.
    2. Start under the jaw and "milk" the big muscle down the throat on each side of the neck, *TOWARDS THE HEART.*
    3. Start just behind the ears and "milk" downward towards the shoulders. Each time move closer toward the spinal column. This can relieve headaches and muscle tension.
    4. Fast stroke seven-ten times towards the heart every 10-15 minutes until relief occurs, in any area that is symptomatic.

HOW YOUR LYMPHATIC SYSTEM PROTECTS YOUR HEALTH:

Your body is constantly in the process of taking in nutrients and eliminating toxic wastes through the following series of events:

- Through the capillaries flow blood that is 91 percent water, oxygen, nutrients, and three blood proteins (albumin, globulin, and fibrinogen). The blood proteins hold the water in the capillaries, as the oxygen and nutrients go through tiny pores to nourish the nearby tightly packed cells.

-White blood cells circulate among those packed cells protecting you from bacteria and viruses, and the lymphatic system carries away any remaining toxins and wastes.

IN THIS PERFECTLY FUNCTIONING SYSTEM, YOUR HEALTH IS MAINTAINED AND PROTECTED. SO WHY ARE SO MANY PEOPLE STRUGGLING WITH HEALTH?

- The pores in the capillaries become **enlarged** from drugs and/or stress. Drugs are being used in epidemic proportions, but even if you do not take any drugs, no one in modern America can escape stress. Stress can come from emotional, financial, relationship or career issues; polluted electromagnetic energy in the atmosphere; total chemical environment; nutritional imbalances, dehydration, or build up of toxic wastes in the body. Stress from any cause allows the smallest of the blood proteins (albumin) to pass through the enlarged capillary pores; with its magnetic attraction to water, the albumin brings water with it, surrounding the cells. Cells, separated with proteins and water, are unable to correctly receive oxygen and nutrients. This is the beginning of degenerative changes in the cells that can lead to symptoms and disease.

- A slow moving lymphatic system is not always able to keep up with pulling off the water and proteins; when this condition builds up in any body area, you can experience local symptoms.

HOW DO YOU PROTECT YOUR LYMPHATICS?

1. Use drugs only in an acute, emergency, or medical condition (like insulin or thyroid) when nothing else will protect your health or life.

2. Learn how to cope with daily stress and build self-esteem.

3. Drink eight glasses of water daily, *unless otherwise indicated by an existing medical condition.*

4. Do "bouncing" type exercise 15 minutes once or twice daily.

5. Recommend you purchase *THE GOLDEN SEVEN PLUS ONE* by C. Samuel West (refer to reference list).

[] [] [] [] [] []

ANOTHER FORM OF ENERGY - MAGNETISM

As a health "student", one value you should get from this book is exposure to many different subjects that affect health. Our modern society has polluted or reduced our exposure to the natural balance of nature.

THE AVERAGE PERSON IS LOW IN ENVIRONMENTAL ELECTROMAGNETIC INTAKE DUE TO THE EARTH'S MAGNETIC FIELD BEING POLLUTED. POWER LINES, TELEVISION, MICROWAVES, RADAR, MODERN LIVING IN STEEL BUILDINGS, CARS, PLANES, TRAINS, BUSES, AND SUBWAYS DEPRIVE US OF REGULAR EXPOSURE TO ELECTROMAGNETIC FORCE.

Every atom, molecule, cell, tissue and organ in our body resonates, or vibrates at its own particular frequency. That body frequency NATURALLY vibrates to, and connects with the earth's energy. This *combination* of energy can occur in every cell, organ and system of our body. It alters the rate of cellular activity, and the chemical processes that effect overall changes in our body.

> *The same body effects can be "created" by applying a magnetic field which performs in the same way. It only takes a very low intensity magnetic field to effect chemical reactions that have a biological effect on our body. There are two main types of magnetism:*
>
> > *- A temporary magnetic field puts out a magnetic field only while electricity is flowing through coils of wire by continually reversing the poles. Changing the direction of a magnetic field induces an electromagnetic force (EMF), producing electrical energy. This can cause cellular chaos, and can create problems as we surround our lives with more and more electrical products. This*

is why you will read articles on not sleeping with electric blankets, or on heated waterbeds.

- Permanent magnetism follows a continuous closed path which travels from North pole to South pole. This is not hazardous because the magnetic field does not change... North and South do not reverse positions causing chaos. Magnetic therapy is a respected medical approach elsewhere in the world, but this country concentrates on more profitable drugs and surgery. The noticeable value of improved circulation with permanent magnetism will benefit any situation like sleep problems, pain, stiffness, and injury.

Books are available in health food stores on magnetic therapy. Catalogs and products are available from the following sources: Mid-American Marketing, PO Box 124, Eaton, OH 45320 (800-922-1744); Family Health News, 800-284-6263; NIKKEN Magnetic Products have local distributors in most areas, or call Nancy Rosenberg (1-410-356-7600).

☐ ☐ ☐ ☐ ☐ ☐

THE IMPORTANCE OF "THE MEANING OF LIFE"

Discussion on the fundamentals of health would not be complete without some reference to THE MEANING OF LIFE. The most primal and basic human need is the need for meaning. Satisfy the meaning of existence for you, and you will make better choices to protect the new found quality of life. The meaning of your life is a very private matter, and so should be your right to search in your own way.

Do not lose your personal power. *HEALTH METAMORPHOSIS* and other health books are part of the exciting adventure in learning about personal development on all levels of physical, emotional, mental, and spiritual. Power is spelled **COMMITMENT**, and that means commitment to:

- personal growth
- personal contribution to mankind

IMPROVED HEALTH WILL FOLLOW AS SURELY AS DAY FOLLOWS NIGHT.

[] [] [] [] [] []

CONGRATULATIONS TO THOSE WHO HAVE COMPLETED THE LAST FIVE CHAPTERS. THIS QUOTE BY AN UNKNOWN WRITER MAY FIT THE WAY YOU FEEL:

"WE HAVE NOT SUCCEEDED IN ANSWERING ALL YOUR PROBLEMS. THE ANSWERS WE HAVE FOUND ONLY SERVE TO RAISE A WHOLE SET OF NEW QUESTIONS. IN SOME WAYS WE FEEL WE ARE AS CONFUSED AS EVER, BUT WE BELIEVE WE ARE CONFUSED ON A HIGHER LEVEL, AND ABOUT MORE IMPORTANT THINGS."

THE ROAD TO HEALTH BECOMES EASIER THROUGH EDUCATION

. . . read on for a few final comments. . .

SUMMARY

METAMORPHOSIS...THE NEW "YOU" EMERGES

"...let us run with endurance the race that is set before us."
Hebrews 12:1

YOU are responsible for your well-being. WELLNESS is as much a state of mind as it is being free of disease. As you live by health promoting standards, the frustrations of life that may once have seemed overwhelming, can now be dealt with as minor annoyances. You have now achieved the ability to control your health, rather than be controlled by your illnesses.

For me, graduation from the "school of health" was the day I climbed to 9,795 foot Eagle Cap Peak in northeastern Oregon. The 40 miles I hiked in six days would have been achievement enough considering my medical history. However, climbing a mountain that just a few years earlier seemed an impossible dream, became an exhilarating highlight in my life. If I could do that hike. . .what else could I do? Each accomplishment produced the energy needed to stretch into new directions . . .with new goals. . .and new hope for the future.

[] [] [] [] [] []

Being a health success story can be another kind of challenge. . .in communication. You have all you can handle learning and applying new knowledge to improve YOUR health, so don't take on the health problems of people around you. Most people do not appreciate being told that what is helping you will be the best thing for them, as well. *ONLY* when they are motivated because of their own illness, or are impressed by your good health, will they be willing to make different choices in their lives. Take care of your own health. . .teach through EXAMPLE! People want to listen when they *ask* what you are doing to improve your health.

Not everyone is willing or able to be strict with their health routine all the time. MODERATION is the key! If you do not have adverse reactions, you may choose to occasionally enjoy a treat socially that is not a perfect health recommendation. Sensible social treats may keep you from feeling deprived, and keep you health-oriented at other times. Remember, **you make or break your health at home**, where you should eat most of your meals. If you eat out a lot, learn to be more selective.

Heredity and aging get the blame for far too much illness today. Many problems are self-inflicted through poor dietary and habit choices, and through overzealous supplement efforts that create body imbalances. When you have symptoms, realize your body is telling you there are problems. Learn to *TUNE IN TO BODY LANGUAGE*. Access how your symptoms may be presently due to neglecting one or more of the EIGHT LAWS OF WELLNESS. As you make changes and your health improves, you will gain confidence from the miracles that can be experienced through your efforts. You will want to expand your knowledge to protect health naturally. Learning ways to protect your health, so you feel well each day, becomes your new hobby.

Your new hobby is not without challenges. Every health suggestion that comes out in print is enthusiastically presented as the answer in achieving wellness. Conflicting opinions in many books, and a fever for detailed options have led to confusion and frustration. It is understandable why some people refuse to get involved with their own health management. When we do make a choice, it often is oversimplified from reading an article like *THINK ZINC*. It does not follow that all you have to do for wellness is to take zinc supplements. Relying solely on your doctor to deal with chronic illness is not the answer either. The answer lies in BALANCE. Live by the COMMON SENSE laws that allow the body to work at optimum performance, or heal itself if possible.

In the coming months you will hear a lot of comments about the harmful effects of too many vitamins. It will draw your attention away from the real issues at hand: the over-medication of people, needless surgery, thousands of worthless drugs, poor health statistics, deterioration of health in our country, the run-a-round from specialist to specialist, and the effort that is being made to prevent people from being part of their own medical treatment plan. DISEASE. . .NOT HEALTH. . .IS BIG BUSINESS!!! We do need to take supplements with knowledge, but the damage from supplement abuse does not begin to compare to the damage from long term drug abuse for chronic problems. Doctors spend years learning the immense field of medicine. All of us have been helped at one time or another by a compassionate doctor. But, nutrition and the principles of wellness are largely ignored in medical school. Many foreign countries are years ahead of the United States in making health products and anti-aging techniques, readily available to their people.

[] [] [] [] [] []

A **summary** on the *principles of wellness* would not be complete without listing these highlights that should be top priority in your quest for well being:

* The more you stick to NATURAL WHOLE FOODS like Spirulina, Blue-Green Algae, Bee Pollen, and Barley Green rather than chemical FRACTIONS in multiple formulas, the more likely you are to achieve the results you desire.

* Live in conformity with the body's circadian rhythm; have a bowel elimination and eat light before noon.

* Raw and unprocessed foods best provide the nutrients your body needs to perform it's many functions. Our low intake of essential fatty acids that are deficient in processed food, is a major contributing factor in many common diseases.

* Reduce red meat and dairy products; better yet, eliminate them except for social situations.

* When chlorine combines with the natural organic matter in the water, volatile pollutants are formed (like chloroform) that can cause disease. An inexpensive shower filter can protect the skin from the toxins created by chlorinated water. Drinking water should be distilled or filtered.

* Fitness can be gained or lost in a 28 day period. Any daily exercise must include a choice that moves the lymphatic system.

* You should test your urine and saliva pH once a month for the rest of your life! **Mark it on your calendar; this is too important to forget.**

* Minerals are easily lost in the typical American diet. Minerals are the catalysts in the chemical reactions that go on in our bodies every day. Minerals like calcium, magnesium, potassium, and sodium are "electrolytes" that transmit electrical nerve impulses. Unprocessed solar or sun-evaporated seasalt is like a tonic for electrolyte balance; or well absorbed natural liquid minerals.

* Supplementing Q10 provides the raw material needed to activate intracellular energy. Q10 is produced in the liver. However, pH imbalance, poor digestion, and a liver stressed from modern day abuse reduces the production of this critical nutrient.

* The body's immune system is too often stretched to the breaking point. Supplements with antioxidants like Vitamins A, C, E, Superoxide Dismutase (SOD), and Selenium help fight off the damage produced by modern day living.

* Besides the recommendations for physical health, you need to connect with your spiritual beliefs, and let the direction you get from your Creator guide you to bring out your strengths, and *turn your lights on.*

* Start every day, first thing in the morning with a *positive attitude* and your *game plan.* You should now be ready to work on your *life wish.* **KEEP FOCUSED!!!**

> "I EXPECT TO PASS THROUGH THIS WORLD BUT ONCE. ANY GOOD THEREFORE THAT I CAN DO, OR ANY KINDNESS OR ABILITIES THAT I CAN SHOW TO ANY FELLOW CREATURE, LET ME DO IT NOW. LET ME NOT DEFER OR NEGLECT IT, FOR I SHALL NOT PASS THIS WAY AGAIN."
>   - William Penn

THIS IS YOUR LIFE...
IT IS NOT A REHEARSAL...
MAKE THE START OF EACH DAY SPECIAL!

"IF WE DID ALL THE THINGS WE ARE CAPABLE OF DOING, WE WOULD LITERALLY ASTONISH OURSELVES."

- Thomas Edison

[] [] [] [] [] []

It is sensible to practice the *PRINCIPLES OF HEALTH*, and prevent disease rather than to treat all the individual symptoms. Since the body is an interrelated system, it is important to treat *THE WHOLE BODY AT ONE TIME*, and not just a single area of concern. Even some health-oriented books support separate body areas by dealing with individual subjects, like nutrition in one book, elimination in another, exercise in another, and personal development in still another. THE BODY SHOULD BE TREATED AS A UNIT. . .SIMPLY, AND WITH BACK-TO-BASICS RECOMMENDATIONS. *HEALTH METAMORPHOSIS* has attempted to teach you the importance of the interrelation between all levels of physical, emotional, mental, and spiritual!

Wellness does not have to be a difficult subject. Learn how to deal with tension and stress through **positive thinking**. Eat food that is *capable* of providing high quality **nutrition**. Consume chemical and parasite free **water**. Be conscious of good **digestion** principles. Help your body **eliminate waste** products at a speed that allows cells to function at peak performance. **Exercise** to *ENJOY LIFE* and promote a healthy circulatory and lymphatic system. This all adds up to COMMON SENSE! DON'T GET LOST IN DETAILS. No given day is a test of all your knowledge implemented perfectly. Relax. . .enjoy your learning experience. Take *pride* in learning how to take responsibility for your health. Make sensible choices. . take care of your body. . .and your body will take care of you.

[] [] [] [] [] []

TO MAINTAIN WELLNESS, EXPAND KNOWLEDGE ON:

POSITIVE THINKING
NUTRITION
DIGESTION
ELIMINATION
EXERCISE

USING THE FOLLOWING PRINCIPLES ON A REGULAR BASIS:

> *ROTATION*
> *MODERATION*
> *BALANCE*
> *COMMON SENSE*

PRACTICING THE EIGHT LAWS OF WELLNESS ON A REGULAR BASIS:

> *WATER*
> *TRACE MINERALS*
> *ESSENTIAL FATTY ACIDS*
> *pH BALANCE*
> *CONTROL OF CANDIDA YEAST AND PARASITES*
> *ELIMINATION*
> *EXERCISE WITH OXYGEN*
> *STRESS MANAGEMENT*

[] [] [] [] [] []

LOOK INTO A MIRROR AND SAY, "I AM WORTHY OF FEELING HEALTHY IN MY BODY AND FEELING GOOD ABOUT MYSELF!" Consider getting color draped, and adding the energy of the best colors for your complexion to your new enthusiasm for life. Introducing exciting color in your life means introducing energy!

Our selection of color is an expression of our acceptance or rejection of ourselves. If a person projects themselves as successful, and if their surroundings are bright, they will carry that energy into the day's activities. Color has a powerful influence on our health from the energy of red, yellow and orange, to the mellow blue, turquoise and purple, and the neutral greens. The more creatively we use color in our food, clothing, and environment, the more natural energy we create to help us develop physically, mentally, and spiritually. Color is the essence of the vital force all around us.

[] [] [] [] [] []

So, dear reader, we have reached the end of a pleasant journey together. You've come a long way in knowledge since you first opened this book. As you close the back cover, you will open a door to the rest of your life. *HEALTH METAMORPHOSIS* will always be on your library shelf, to freshen your memory, or just remind you that learning is fun. You can now develop your own self-confidence, dedication to your well-being, and an enthusiasm for life that will make daily decisions easier. Through your **metamorphosis** you will discover challenges and make plans that will give new meaning to your life. I congratulate you on completing this book. . .you are worth it!

HAVE A GREAT LIFE!!!

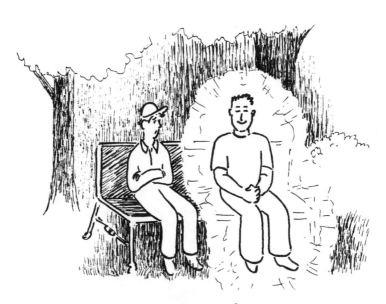

I take it you're using those
ALTERNATIVE MEDICINES again !?

RECOMMENDED BOOKS

THE FOLLOWING BOOKS ARE **HIGHLY RECOMMENDED:**

* **Alternative Medicine - The Definitive Guide** - compiled by the Burton Goldberg Group - 1994 - Future Medicine Publishing, Inc., 5009 Pacific Hwy. E, Suite 6, Fife, WA 98424
* **Apple Cider Vinegar, Miracle Health System** - by Paul and Patricia Bragg - c.1996 - Health Science, Box 7, Santa Barbara, CA 93102; 1-800-446-1990; http://www.bragg.com
* **Don't Eat the Yellow Snow** - Gary A. Martin, D.Sc., Ph.D - 1987 - Martin Health Systems; 1-800-321-6917
* **Dr. Whitaker's Guide To Natural Healing** - Julian Whitaker, M.D. - 1995 - Prima Publishing, P.O. Box 1260BK, Rocklin, CA 95677; 1-916-632-4440
* **If It's Going To Be, It's Up To Me** - Robert H. Schuller - 1997 - Harper Collins; 1-800-9POWER9
* **The Biochemic Handbook** - 1976 - Formur, Inc., 4200 Laclede Ave., St. Louis, MO 63108
* **The Chemistry of Man** - Bernard Jensen, Ph.D. - 1983 - Bernard Jensen Enterprises, 24360 Old Wagon Road, Escondido, CA 92027
* **The Cure For All Diseases** - Hulda Regehr Clark, Ph.D., N.D. - 1995 - Promotion Publishing, 3368F Governor Drive, Suite 144, San Diego, CA 92122; 1-800-231-1776
* **The Golden Seven Plus One (Conquer Disease with Eight Keys to Health, Beauty, and Peace)** - C. Samuel West, D.N., N.D. - 1981 - Samuel Publishing Co., P.O. Box 1051, Orem, UT 84059; 1-800-975-0123
* **The Yeast Connection** - William G. Crook, M.D. - 1983 - Professional Books, P.O. Box 3246, Jackson, TN 38303
* **Your Body's Many Cries For Water** - F. Batmanghelidj, M.D. - 1995 - Global Health Solutions, 2146 Kings Garden Way, Falls Church, VA 22043; 1-703-848-2333

THE FOLLOWING BOOKS ARE **EXCELLENT** ADDITIONS TO YOUR WELLNESS LIBRARY. ANY BOOKSTORE CAN ORDER FOR YOU:

* **Acid & Alkaline** - Herman Aihara - 1986 - George Ohsawa Macrobiotic Foundation, 1511 Robinson Street, Oroville, CA 95965
* **Alkalize or Die** - Theodore A. Baroody, N.D., D.C., Ph.D. Nutrition, C.N.C. - 1991 - Eclectic Press, 205 Pigeon Street, Waynesville, NC 28786; 1-800-566-1522
* **Dr. Abravanel's Body Type Diet and Lifetime Nutrition Plan** - Eliot D. Abravanel, M.D. - 1983 - Bantam Books, Inc., New York, NY 10103
* **Dr. Christopher's Three Day Cleanse, Mucusless Diet, and Herbal Combinations** - John Christopher - 1996 - Christopher Publications 1-800-372-8255
* **How to Survive the Loss of a Love** - Melba Colgrove, Ph.D., Harold H. Bloomfield, M.D., Peter McWilliams - 1991 - Bantam Books, New York
* **The Milk Book** - William Campbell Douglass, M.D. - 1994 - Second Opinion Publishing, P. O. Box 467939, Atlanta, GA 31146-7939; 1-800-728-2288
* **Physician's Reference Notebook** - William McGarey, M.D. - 1996 - A.R.E. Press, P.O. Box 595, Virginia Beach, VA 23451; 1-800-723-1112
* **Pocket Manual of Homeopathic Materia Medica** - William Boericke, M.D. - 1927 - Boericke & Runyon, Philadelphia, PA (Source for Homeopathic Remedy information)
* **The Cure For All Cancers** - Hulda Regehr Clark, Ph.D., N.D. - 1993 - Promotion Publishing, 3368F Governor Drive, Suite 144, San Diego, CA 92122; 1-800-231-1776
* **The Essiac Report** - Richard Thomas - 1993 - The Alternative Treatment Information Network, 1244 Ozeta Terrace, Los Angeles, CA 90069; 1-310-278-6611
* **The Herb Book** - John Lust, N.D., D.B.M. - 1974 - Bantam Books, Inc., New York, NY 10103
* **The New Possibility Thinkers Bible** - Robert H. Schuller and Paul David Dunn - 1996 - Thomas Nelson Publishers; 1-800-976-9379

RECOMMENDED REFERENCES:

Aloe Vera - cold-pressed, whole leaf, and 10X concentrate can be purchased from Bliss Associates, 1-888-432-5477

Arbonne natural cosmetics - 1-800-ARBONNE

Celtic Sea Salt, extra fine - HomeCure, Inc., Scottsdale, AZ 85260; 1-800-559-2873. Product and book also available from The Grain and Salt Society, P.O. Box DD, Magalia, CA 95954

Chi Machine - manufactured by Sun Harmony (HTE USA, Inc., Plainview, NY) - distributed by Bethany 40 Wellness Center, 10176 Route 40 West, Suite 107, Ellicott City, MD 21042; 1-410-418-5969. Business hours: Mon. & Thur. 11AM-7PM; Tues., Wed., Fri. 10AM-6PM, EST.

Discover Homeopathy - catalogue of homeopathic products and books 1-800-359-9051

Flora, Inc. - for Flor-Essence, Elderberry Cleanse, and Herbal Iron; 1-800-498-3610

N.E.E.D.S. Catalog (environmental products) - 1-800-634-1380

Pines International (organic products) - 1-800-MY-PINES

Royal Body Care, Inc./Light Force - 10575 Newkirk, Suite 780, Dallas, TX 75220-2327; 1-800-722-0444; under ID# 920010984

Sea Farine (a nutritional intestinal cleanser product) - Sea Farine, 1641 Warner Ave., McLean, VA 22121; 1-703-356-2672

Walnut Acres Organic Farms - Penns Creek, Pa; 1-800-433-3998

ORDERING INFORMATION

For additional copies of this book, please call:

Kendall/Hunt Customer Service
1-800-228-0810

Discounts for quantity orders:

12-24 books	10%
24-50 books	20%
over 50 books	30%

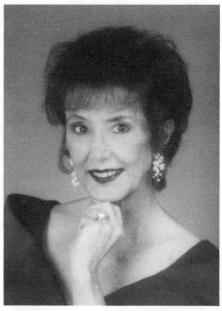
© 1997 Glamour Shots ®

ABOUT THE AUTHOR

THE PROFESSIONAL:
Dori Luneski has been a leader in the health field for over 30 years. She worked in a holistic health clinic for 12 years, as a rehabilitation nurse for two years, and a psychiatric nurse for six years. That background, and her naturopathic doctor degree, gives her insight into all aspects of wellness and stress management.

THE SPEAKER:
Dori is a trained professional in public speaking through National Speakers Association, and delivers speeches, seminars, and courses on stress management, and self-responsibility in health care. She is a one-stop source of information on all levels of physical, emotional and mental health.

THE PERSONAL HEALTH SUCCESS STORY:
For 20 years, Dori was chemically ill and physically and emotionally weak; at age 45 she was bed-ridden. Now at age 63, people marvel at her vitality, energy and enthusiasm; and eagerly listen to her powerful presentations on how to protect the qualtiy of life. Her book, *HEALTH METAMORPHOSIS* shares the success of her efforts.